Anti-Inflammatory
Diet Cookbook for
Beginners

2000 Days

of Quick & Easy Recipes to Lose Weight, Detox Your Body, and Regain Well-Being by Harnessing the Power of the Anti-Inflammatory Diet

Dorothy Williams

Contents

Chapter 6: Fish & Seafood Recipes 56

Chapter 7: Vegetarian Recipes 67

Chapter 8: Wraps & Sandwiches Recipes 78

Chapter 9: Snacks & Appetizer Recipes 87

Chapter 10: Dessert Recipes 95

30 Days Meal Plan 104

Conversion Chart 106

Conclusion 108

Introduction

What is Anti-Inflammatory Diet?

An anti-inflammatory diet can be a powerful tool for improving health and preventing chronic diseases. It focuses on foods that have been proven to reduce inflammation in the body, such as fruits, vegetables, whole grains, lean proteins, nuts and healthy fats. Eating this way provides essential nutrients needed to lessen inflammation and help the body repair itself naturally. This type of dietary intervention also brings additional benefits such as increased energy levels, improved digestion, decreased stress levels and better overall well-being.

The anti-inflammatory diet is becoming increasingly popular among health-conscious individuals. It emphasizes eating whole, unprocessed foods that have been naturally grown, and restricts the intake of food known to trigger inflammation. Examples of foods suggested by the anti-inflammatory diet include fruits, vegetables, nuts, seeds, fish and other seafood, whole grains such as quinoa and oats, herbs, spices, healthy fats like olive oil and avocado and green tea. On the otherhand it excludes processed meats like hot dogs or deli slices; fried foods; refined grains like white flour and white rice; sugary drinks; trans fats like margarine; and processed olive oils such as corn oil or cottonseed oil. By avoiding these items known to worsen inflammation in the body and instead opting for whole-nutrition sources such as fresh produce, this diet offers many potential health benefits.

Symptoms of Chronic Inflammation

Chronic inflammation is a subtle, slowly-progressing condition that can wreak havoc on the body and ultimately lead to more serious illnesses. It manifests itself differently in each person, but many of the symptoms are the same. Fatigue, pain, digestive issues and sleep difficulties are all common warning signs of chronic inflammation. If any of these symptoms continue over a long period of time without improvement, it is best to consult with a doctor to discuss further treatment options. Left untreated, chronic inflammation can have severe effects on health and well-being.

Signs and Symptoms of Chronic Inflammation:

Chronic inflammation is a long-term inflammatory process that can have a range of symptoms, many of which may be mild or even unnoticeable. Some of the most common signs and symptoms of chronic inflammation include:

1. Fatigue: Constant fatigue or exhaustion can be one of the first signs that you are experiencing chronic inflammation due to an underlying medical condition.
2. Joint Pain: While joint pain is often associated with injury or arthritis, it can also be a sign of long-term inflammation in the body.
3. Redness and Swelling: Redness, swelling and warmth in affected areas are classic signs of acute inflammation but can also occur due to chronic inflammation.
4. Fever/Chills: A fever is your body's response to infection as well as its natural defense against invaders. The same can be true when your body is trying to fight off underlying chronic inflammation. It may cause episodes of fever and chills accompanied by other flu-like symptoms such as nausea and vomiting.
5. Weight Fluctuations: Unexplained weight fluctuations are another sign that your body may be battling underlying inflammatory processes within it. Weight loss or gain could indicate an imbalance in energy expenditure caused by immune system responses related to chronic inflammation.
6. Skin Changes: Skin changes, such as red patches, rashes, hives, acne, or psoriasis could signal underlying systemic issues related to chronic inflammation in the body.
7. Digestive Issues: Many digestive issues such as abdominal pain, bloating, diarrhea and constipation can all be linked to chronic inflammatory conditions such as irritable bowel syndrome (IBS).
8. Poor Sleep Quality: Poor sleep quality is connected with a number of health problems including depression and anxiety disorders but can also indicate an imbalance caused by underlying inflammation levels in the body.
9. Headaches/Migraines: Chronic headaches can also indicate more serious issues like brain fog or neurological disorders but they may be linked to ongoing systemic inflammatory processes too.
10. Depression/Anxiety Disorders: Recent studies have shown how mental health issues like depression and anxiety disorders could actually be manifesting from systemic levels of ongoing inflammation within the body rather than just being psychological phenomena alone.

How to Prevent and Control Inflammation

Inflammation is the body's natural response to injury and infection, but when it becomes chronic, it can lead to a variety of health problems. Fortunately, there are several strategies that you can use to both prevent and control inflammation, helping you stay healthy and active.

1. Eat an Anti-Inflammatory Diet: Eating a well-balanced diet is one of the best ways to reduce inflammation in the body. Foods that are high in antioxidants, omega-3 fatty acids, and fiber can help reduce inflammation. These include fruits and vegetables such as apples, oranges, spinach, kale and berries; healthy fats like olive oil and avocados; nuts; legumes; fish; and whole grains.

2. Exercise Regularly: Regular physical activity helps to reduce overall inflammation in the body by promoting circulation and reducing stress levels. Aim for at least 30 minutes of exercise each day, focusing on activities that you enjoy such as walking, swimming, biking, or light weightlifting.

3. Manage Stress Levels: Stress has been linked to increased levels of inflammation in the body due to its effect on hormones like cortisol and adrenaline. To manage stress levels naturally try practices such as yoga, meditation or mindfulness exercises. Journaling can also be beneficial for managing stress by allowing you to express your thoughts and feelings around stressful events or experiences.

4. 4. Get Enough Rest: Restful sleep is essential for helping the body recover from daily stressors and reducing inflammation levels in the body. Aim for 7-9 hours of quality sleep each night by establishing a bedtime routine that includes no screens or stimulating activities before bedtime and winding down for an hour or two before turning out the lights for the night.

5. Take Anti-Inflammatory Supplements: Natural supplements such as turmeric, ginger root extract, omega 3 fatty acids (fish oil), vitamin D3 and probiotics can help reduce inflammation in the body when taken regularly over time. However, it's important to consult with your healthcare provider before starting any supplements as they may interact with other medications you are taking or have adverse effects on certain medical conditions you may have.

6. Avoid Processed Foods: Processed foods contain added sugars which can fuel inflammatory responses in the body over time so try avoiding them as much as possible since they offer little nutritional value anyway!

7. Drink plenty of water: Proper hydration is key for helping to flush out toxins from your system which can lead to increased levels of inflammation so make sure you're drinking enough water throughout the day!

8. Consume healthy fats & oils: Fats & oils found naturally in foods like avocado nuts seeds olives coconut oil etc. Help regulate inflammatory responses within our bodies so we must consume them regularly throughout our diets!

Anti-Inflammatory Diet Food List

Eating an anti-inflammatory diet is essential for living a healthy lifestyle and managing inflammation in the body. An anti-inflammatory diet helps to reduce inflammation levels in the body which can cause chronic health issues such as arthritis, allergies, autoimmune disorders, heart disease, diabetes, and other illnesses. A well-balanced anti-inflammatory diet consists of fresh fruits and vegetables, lean proteins, complex carbohydrates, healthy fats, probiotic foods and spices that are known to have anti-inflammatory properties. Here is an extensive list of food options to incorporate into your anti-inflammatory meal plan.

Fruits:

Fruits are a great source of vitamins, minerals and antioxidants that help reduce inflammation and boost the immune system. Some beneficial fruits for an anti-inflammatory diet include apples, oranges, pears, berries (blueberries & strawberries), kiwi fruit, pineapple, bananas and grapefruit. Eating these fruits will provide essential nutrients like vitamin C and potassium that are needed for optimal health.

Vegetables:

Vegetables are packed with vitamins and minerals which make them some of the best foods to consume on an anti-inflammatory diet. Some recommended vegetables include leafy greens (spinach & kale), bell peppers (red & green), broccoli & cauliflower (cruciferous veggies), zucchini & squash (summer veggies) asparagus & artichoke hearts (non-starch veggies). Incorporating a variety of these vegetables into your meals will provide plenty of fiber as well as key nutrients that can help combat inflammation in the body.

Proteins:

Getting enough protein is important on any type of diet including an anti-inflammatory one. Protein sources for this type of eating plan include fish such as salmon or tuna which contain omega 3 fatty acids that fight inflammation in the body as well as lean cuts of meat such as chicken or turkey breast which are high in vitamins B6 & B12 needed for immunity health. Other sources include tofu, tempeh or seitan if you're following a plant-based diet or eggs from cage-free hens if you're consuming dairy products. All these protein sources should be organic when it is possible for maximum nutritional content

Complex Carbohydrates:

It's important to get enough energy from carbohydrates on any type of diet including an anti-inflammatory one. Complex carbohydrates provide sustained energy throughout the day without causing spikes in blood sugar levels which can contribute to inflammation in the body so they're perfect for this type of eating plan. Whole grains like quinoa, brown rice, oats or millet are ideal while legumes such as lentils, beans, chickpeas or black-eyed peas should also be eaten regularly due to their high fiber content. Potatoes may also be consumed but should be limited because they have a higher glycemic index than other carbohydrates.

Healthy Fats

Healthy fats are essential for proper hormone balance and overall wellness so it's important to get enough on an anti-inflammatory diet. Sources include avocados, nuts & seeds like almonds, walnuts, flaxseed, chia seed etc., olive oil or coconut oil when cooking at low temperatures and fatty fish such as salmon which provides omega-3 fatty acids needed by our bodies. All these fats should be unprocessed cold pressed oils or organic whenever possible.

Probiotic Foods

Probiotics act as natural antibiotics by providing good bacteria to our bodies helping rebalance gut flora which can lead to increased immunity levels thus reducing inflammation caused by bad bacteria. Examples include yogurt, kefir, kombucha tea or fermented vegetables such sauerkraut, kimchi etc., all made from raw organic ingredients whenever possible.

Anti-Inflammatory Spices

Spices contain powerful compounds called polyphenols that fight against free radicals preventing cellular damage leading to inflammation. Commonly used spices for this purpose include turmeric, ginger root powder cloves nutmeg cayenne powder cinnamon cardamom garlic oregano rosemary basil parsley thyme etc., all making delicious additions to meals while providing amazing health benefits.

Get the Best out from your Anti-Inflammatory Diet

Eating an anti-inflammatory diet is essential for promoting overall health and wellness. Amongst its benefits, such a diet can help boost immunity, reduce cholesterol levels and improve digestion. When done correctly, this approach to eating can also help with weight management. To get the most out of your anti-inflammatory diet, try to focus on natural foods like fruits and vegetables that are rich in antioxidants. Additionally, opt for lean protein sources like fish or skinless poultry along with whole grains and legumes for healthy carbohydrates. Furthermore, be sure to include good fats from nuts, seeds and olives in your meals. By making such choices when it comes to fueling your body you can enjoy all the benefits that come with an anti-inflammatory lifestyle.

CHAPTER 1:
Smoothie Recipes

Pineapple Smoothie

Serves: 2 individuals
Preparation Time: 10 minutes
Ingredients:

- 1 cup frozen pineapple
- 1 large ripe banana, peeled and sliced
- ½ tablespoon fresh ginger, peeled and chopped
- ¼ teaspoon ground turmeric
- 1 cup unsweetened almond milk
- ½ cup fresh carrot juice
- 1 tablespoon fresh lemon juice

Directions:

1. In a high-powered blender, add all ingredients and pulse until creamy and smooth.
2. Transfer the smoothie into 2 glasses and serve immediately.

Nutritional Information per Serving:
Calories: 140
Fat: 2.2g
Net Carbohydrates: 27g
Carbohydrates: 31.4g
Fiber: 4.4g
Sugar: 18g
Protein: 2.1g
Sodium: 113mg

Pineapple & Orange Smoothie

Serves: 2 individuals
Preparation Time: 10 minutes
Ingredients:

- 1 fresh orange, peeled and chopped
- 2 cups fresh pineapple, chopped
- 1 (1-inch) piece fresh ginger, peeled and chopped
- 1 frozen banana, peeled and sliced
- 1 teaspoon ground turmeric
- 1 tablespoon chia seeds
- 1½ cup unsweetened almond milk
- ¼ cup ice cubes

Directions:

1. In a high-powered blender, add all ingredients and pulse until creamy and smooth.
2. Transfer the smoothie into 2 glasses and serve immediately.

Nutritional Information per Serving:
Calories: 226
Fat: 4.5g
Net Carbohydrates: 41.4g
Carbohydrates: 49.7g
Fiber: 8.3g
Sugar: 32.1g
Protein: 4g
Sodium: 138mg

Papaya & Pineapple Smoothie

Serves: 2 individuals
Preparation Time: 10 minutes
Ingredients:

- 2 cups pineapple, peeled and chopped
- 1½ cups papaya, peeled and chopped
- 2-3 dates, pitted
- 1½ cups coconut water
- ¼ cup ice cubes

Directions:

1. In a high-powered blender, add all ingredients and pulse until creamy and smooth.
2. Transfer the smoothie into 2 glasses and serve immediately.

Nutritional Information per Serving
Calories: 151
Fat: 0.7g
Net Carbohydrates: 31.4g
Carbohydrates: 37.2g
Fiber: 5.8g
Sugar: 27.8g
Protein: 2.5g
Sodium: 197mg

Peach Smoothie

Serves: 2 individuals
Preparation Time: 10 minutes
Ingredients:

- 1 frozen banana, peeled and chopped
- 2 cups frozen peaches, pitted and chopped
- ½ teaspoon ground ginger
- ½ teaspoon chia seeds
- 1 teaspoon ground turmeric
- 1 teaspoon ground cinnamon
- 1 teaspoon organic honey
- 10 ounces unsweetened almond milk

Directions:

1. In a high-powered blender, add all ingredients and pulse until creamy and smooth.
2. Transfer the smoothie into 2 glasses and serve immediately.

Nutritional Information per Serving:
Calories: 156
Fat: 2.9g
Net Carbohydrates: 28.2g
Carbohydrates: 33.7g
Fiber: 5.5g
Sugar: 24.2g
Protein: 2.9g
Sodium: 103mg

Mango & Spinach Smoothie

Serves: 2 individuals
Preparation Time: 10 minutes
Ingredients:

- 2 cups frozen mango, peeled, pitted and chopped

- 3 cups fresh spinach, chopped
- 1 teaspoon ground turmeric
- 1 teaspoon fresh lemon juice
- 1 teaspoon fresh lime juice
- 16 ounces water

Directions:
1. In a high-powered blender, add all ingredients and pulse until creamy and smooth.
2. Transfer the smoothie into 2 glasses and serve immediately.

Nutritional Information per Serving:
Calories: 114
Fat: 0.9g
Net Carbohydrates: 23.2g
Carbohydrates: 27.1g
Fiber: 3.9g
Sugar: 22.8g
Protein: 2.8g
Sodium: 38mg

Orange & Chia Smoothie

Serves: 2 individuals
Preparation Time: 10 minutes
Ingredients:
- 1 orange, peeled, seeded and sliced
- 1 carrot, peeled and chopped
- 1 tablespoon fresh ginger root, peeled and chopped
- 5-10 fresh mint leaves
- 1 tablespoon ground chia seeds
- 1 teaspoon organic honey
- 1 cup spring water
- ½ cup fresh orange juice
- 1 tablespoon fresh lemon juice
- Ice, as required

Directions:
1. In a high-powered blender, add all ingredients and pulse until creamy and smooth.
2. Transfer the smoothie into 2 glasses and serve immediately.

Nutritional Information per Serving
Calories: 114
Fat: 1.6g
Net Carbohydrates: 20.8g
Carbohydrates: 25.4g
Fiber: 4.6g
Sugar: 18.4g
Protein: 2.5g
Sodium: 24mg

Orange & Carrot Smoothie

Serves: 2 individuals
Preparation Time: 10 minutes
Ingredients:
- 1 orange, peeled, seeded and sliced
- 1 carrot, peeled and chopped
- 1 tablespoon fresh ginger root, peeled and chopped
- 5-10 fresh mint leaves

- 1 tablespoon ground chia seeds
- 1 teaspoon organic honey
- 1 cup spring water
- ½ cup fresh orange juice
- 1 tablespoon fresh lemon juice
- Ice, as needed

Directions:
1. In a high-powered blender, add all ingredients and pulse until creamy and smooth.
2. Transfer the smoothie into 2 glasses and serve immediately.

Nutritional Information per Serving:
Calories: 113
Fat: 1.6g
Net Carbohydrates: 20.8g
Carbohydrates: 25.2g
Fiber: 4.4g
Sugar: 18.4g
Protein: 2.4g
Sodium: 23mg

Papaya, Pear & Peach Smoothie

Serves: 2 individuals
Preparation Time: 10 minutes
Ingredients:
- ½ cup pear, peeled, cored and chopped
- ¾ cup peaches, pitted and chopped
- ¾ cup papaya, peeled and chopped
- 1 teaspoon fresh ginger, peeled and chopped
- 2 fresh mint leaves
- ½ cup coconut water
- 1 cup ice, crushed

Directions:
1. In a high-powered blender, add all ingredients and pulse until creamy and smooth.
2. Transfer the smoothie into 2 glasses and serve immediately.

Nutritional Information per Serving:
Calories: 84
Fat: 0.5g
Net Carbohydrates: 16.3g
Carbohydrates: 20.2g
Fiber: 3.9g
Sugar: 15g
Protein: 1.5g
Sodium: 169mg

Blueberry & Cucumber Smoothie

Serves: 2 individuals
Preparation Time: 10 minutes

Ingredients:
- 1½ cups frozen blueberries
- 1 small banana, peeled and sliced
- 1 cup cucumber, peeled and chopped
- 1 tablespoon chia seeds
- 1½ cups water

- ¼ cup ice cubes

Directions:
1. In a high-powered blender, add all ingredients and pulse until creamy and smooth.
2. Transfer the smoothie into 2 glasses and serve immediately.

Nutritional Information per Serving:
Calories: 137
Fat: 1.9g
Net Carbohydrates: 26.9g
Carbohydrates: 32.6g
Fiber: 5.7g
Sugar: 18.9g
Protein: 2.6g
Sodium: 2mg

Strawberry & Beet Smoothie

Serves: 2 individuals
Preparation Time: 10 minutes

Ingredients:
- 2 cups frozen strawberries, pitted and chopped
- 2/3 cup beet, chopped
- 1 teaspoon fresh ginger, peeled and grated
- 1 teaspoon fresh turmeric, peeled and grated
- ½ cup fresh orange juice
- 1 cup unsweetened almond milk

Directions:
1. In a high-powered blender, add all ingredients and pulse until creamy and smooth.
2. Transfer the smoothie into 2 glasses and serve immediately.

Nutritional Information per Serving:
Calories: 126
Fat: 2g
Net Carbohydrates: 21.8g
Carbohydrates: 26.7g
Fiber: 4.9g
Sugar: 18.7g
Protein: 2g
Sodium: 134mg

Strawberry, Apple & Beet Smoothie

Serves: 2 individuals
Preparation Time: 10 minutes
Ingredients:
- 1 cup frozen strawberries, hulled
- 1 beet, peeled and chopped
- 1 apple, peeled, cored and sliced
- 2 Medjool dates, pitted and chopped
- 1 tablespoon extra-virgin coconut oil
- 1½ cups unsweetened almond milk
- ¼ cup ice cubes

Directions:
1. In a high-powered blender, add all ingredients and pulse until creamy and smooth.
2. Transfer the smoothie into 2 glasses and serve immediately.

Nutritional Information per Serving:
Calories: 254
Fat: 10g
Net Carbohydrates: 35.8g
Carbohydrates: 43.4g
Fiber: 7.6g
Sugar: 32.7g
Protein: 2.4g
Sodium: 175mg

Strawberry, Spinach & Celery Smoothie

Serves: 2 individuals
Preparation Time: 10 minutes
Ingredients:
- 1½ cups frozen strawberries
- 2 cups fresh spinach
- 1 cup celery stalk, chopped
- 1 (2-inch) piece fresh ginger, peeled and chopped
- 3 tablespoons hemp protein powder
- 1½ cups filtered water

Directions:
1. In a high-powered blender, add all ingredients and pulse until creamy and smooth.
2. Transfer the smoothie into 2 glasses and serve immediately.

Nutritional Information per Serving:
Calories: 119
Fat: 3.2g
Net Carbohydrates: 9.1g
Carbohydrates: 14.8g
Fiber: 5.7g
Sugar: 8g
Protein: 8.6g
Sodium: 72mg

Berries & Spinach Smoothie

Serves: 2 individuals
Preparation Time: 10 minutes
Ingredients:
- ¾ cup frozen blackberries
- ¾ cup frozen blueberries
- 1 frozen banana, peeled and sliced
- 1 cup fresh baby spinach
- ¼ cup raw walnuts
- 1 teaspoon bee pollen
- 1½ cups unsweetened almond milk

Directions:
1. In a high-powered blender, add all ingredients and pulse until creamy and smooth.
2. Transfer the smoothie into 2 glasses and serve immediately.

Nutritional Information per Serving:
Calories: 242
Fat: 12.6g
Net Carbohydrates: 22.8g
Carbohydrates: 30.6g
Fiber: 7.8g
Sugar: 15.5g
Protein: 7.2g
Sodium: 149mg

Berries & Cottage Cheese Smoothie

Serves: 2 individuals
Preparation Time: 10 minutes
Ingredients:
- 2½ cups frozen mixed berries
- 3 tablespoons unsweetened coconut, shredded
- ¼ cup low-fat cottage cheese
- 1 packet stevia
- 1½ cups coconut water
- ½ cup ice, crushed

Directions:
1. In a high-powered blender, add all ingredients and pulse until creamy and smooth.
2. Transfer the smoothie into 2 glasses and serve immediately.

Nutritional Information per Serving:
Calories: 186
Fat: 4g
Net Carbohydrates: 21.2g
Carbohydrates: 30.1g
Fiber: 8.9g
Sugar: 17.8g
Protein: 6.7g
Sodium: 305mg

Cherry & Blueberry Smoothie

Serves: 2 individuals
Preparation Time: 10 minutes
Ingredients:
- 1½ cups frozen blueberries
- 1½ cups frozen cherries
- ¼ teaspoon ground cinnamon
- ¼ teaspoon ground turmeric
- 1 scoop chocolate protein powder
- 1½ cups filtered water
- ¼ cup ice cubes

Directions:
1. In a high-powered blender, add all ingredients and pulse until creamy and smooth.
2. Transfer the smoothie into 2 glasses and serve immediately.

Nutritional Information per Serving:
Calories: 159
Fat: 0.8g
Net Carbohydrates: 28.4g
Carbohydrates: 33.7g

Fiber: 5.3g
Sugar: 25.6g
Protein: 7.4g
Sodium: 41mg

Cherry & Pineapple Smoothie

Serves: 2 individuals
Preparation Time: 10 minutes

Ingredients:
- 1½ cups pineapple, peeled and chopped
- 1 cup fresh cherries, pitted
- ¼ of beetroot, peeled and chopped
- 1 tablespoon chia seeds
- 1½ cups coconut water
- ¼ cup ice, crushed

Directions:
1. In a high-powered blender, add all ingredients and pulse until creamy and smooth.
2. Transfer the smoothie into 2 glasses and serve immediately.

Nutritional Information per Serving:
Calories: 161
Fat: 1.8g
Net Carbohydrates: 30g
Carbohydrates: 36.7g
Fiber: 6.7g
Sugar: 27.4g
Protein: 3.9g
Sodium: 200mg

Cherry & Kale Smoothie

Serves: 2 individuals
Preparation Time: 10 minutes

Ingredients:
- 2 ripe bananas, peeled and sliced
- 1 cup fresh cherries, pitted
- 2 cups fresh kale, trimmed
- 1 teaspoon fresh ginger, peeled and chopped
- 1 tablespoon chia seeds, soaked for 15 minutes
- ½ teaspoon ground turmeric
- ¼ teaspoon ground cinnamon
- 1½ cups coconut water
- ¼ cup ice cubes

Directions:
1. In a high-powered blender, add all ingredients and pulse until creamy and smooth.
2. Transfer the smoothie into 2 glasses and serve immediately.

Nutritional Information per Serving:
Calories: 238
Fat: 2.1g
Net Carbohydrates: 45.2g
Carbohydrates: 54.4g
Fiber: 9.2g
Sugar: 28.7g
Protein: 6.5g

Sodium: 220mg

Avocado & Kale Smoothie

Serves: 2 individuals
Preparation Time: 10 minutes

Ingredients:

- 2 cups fresh kale, trimmed and chopped
- 1-2 celery stalks, chopped
- ½ of avocado, peeled, pitted and chopped
- 1 (½-inch) piece fresh ginger root, chopped
- 1 (½-inch) piece fresh turmeric root, chopped
- 1½ cups unsweetened coconut milk
- ¼ cup ice cubes

Directions:

1. In a high-powered blender, add all ingredients and pulse until creamy and smooth.
2. Transfer the smoothie into 2 glasses and serve immediately.

Nutritional Information per Serving:

Calories: 364
Fat: 30.3g
Net Carbohydrates: 11.4g
Carbohydrates: 14.5g
Fiber: 3.1g
Sugar: 4.8g
Protein: 4.9g
Sodium: 94mg

Fruit & Veggie Smoothie

Serves: 2 individuals
Preparation Time: 10 minutes

Ingredients:

- ¾ cup pineapple, chopped
- ½ of pear, peeled, cored and chopped
- 1 small avocado, peeled, pitted and chopped
- ½ cup cucumber, peeled and chopped
- 1 cup fresh spinach, chopped
- 1 celery stalk, chopped
- ½ tablespoon fresh dill
- ¼ teaspoon ground turmeric
- 1 piece fresh ginger, peeled
- 1 tablespoon fresh lime juice
- 2 cups water

Directions:

1. In a high-powered blender, add all ingredients and pulse until creamy and smooth.
2. Transfer the smoothie into 2 glasses and serve immediately.

Nutritional Information per Serving:

Calories: 179
Fat: 11.3g
Net Carbohydrates: 14.2g
Carbohydrates: 20.7g
Fiber: 6.5g
Sugar: 10.4g
Protein: 2.4g
Sodium: 25mg

Veggies & Turmeric Smoothie

Serves: 2 individuals
Preparation Time: 10 minutes

Ingredients:
- 1 small avocado, peeled, pitted and chopped
- ½ of green bell pepper, seeded and chopped
- 1 cup fresh baby spinach, chopped
- 1 cup fresh arugula, chopped
- 1 (1-inch) piece fresh turmeric, peeled and grated
- 1 (1-inch) piece fresh ginger, peeled and chopped
- ¾ cup fresh parsley
- Pinch of cayenne powder
- Pinch of salt
- 1½ cups fresh coconut water
- ¼ cup ice cubes

Directions:
1. In a high-powered blender, add all ingredients and pulse until creamy and smooth.
2. Transfer the smoothie into 2 glasses and serve immediately.

Nutritional Information per Serving:
Calories: 174
Fat: 11.8g
Net Carbohydrates: 8.8g
Carbohydrates: 16.2g
Fiber: 7.4g
Sugar: 7g
Protein: 4.1g
Sodium: 298mg

CHAPTER 2:
Breakfast Recipes

Blueberry Smoothie Bowl

Serves: 3 individuals
Preparation Time: 10 minutes

Ingredients:
- 1½ cups frozen blueberries
- ¼ cup unflavored protein powder
- ¼ cup MCT oil
- 2 tablespoons chia seeds
- 1 teaspoon organic vanilla extract
- 4 drops liquid stevia
- 1½ cups unsweetened almond milk

Directions:
1. Add frozen blueberries and remaining ingredients in a high-powered blender and pulse until smooth.
2. Transfer into 3 serving bowls and serve with your favorite topping.

Nutritional Information per Serving
Calories: 198
Fat: 22.4g
Net Carbohydrates: 3.3g
Carbohydrates: 8.1g
Fiber: 4.8g
Sugar: 2g
Protein: 2g
Sodium: 91mg

Fruity Greens Smoothie Bowl

Serves: 2 individuals
Preparation Time: 10 minutes

Ingredients:
- 1 cup fresh strawberries, hulled
- 2 medium ripe bananas, previously sliced and frozen
- ¼ of ripe avocado, peeled, pitted and chopped
- 1 cup fresh spinach
- 1 cup fresh kale, trimmed
- 1 tablespoon flaxseed meal
- 1½ cups unsweetened almond milk

Directions:
1. In a high-powered blender, add strawberries and remaining ingredients and pulse until smooth.
2. Transfer into serving bowls and serve with your favorite topping.

Nutritional Information per Serving:
Calories: 225
Fat: 7.2g
Net Carbohydrates: 32.2g
Carbohydrates: 40.2g
Fiber: 8g
Sugar: 18.1g
Protein: 4.9g
Sodium: 165mg

Fruity Yogurt Bowl

Serves: 2 individuals
Preparation Time: 10 minutes

Ingredients:
- 1 cup fat-free Plain Greek yogurt
- 2 tablespoons Erythritol
- ½ cup peaches, pitted and chopped
- ½ cup fresh raspberries
- ¼ cup fresh blueberries
- ¼ cup fresh cherries, pitted
- 2 tablespoons macadamia nuts, crushed

Directions:
1. In a large-sized bowl, place the yogurt.
2. Add remaining ingredients and gently, stir to blend.
3. Serve immediately.

Nutritional Information per Serving:
Calories: 168
Fat: 6.8g
Net Carbohydrates: 18g
Carbohydrates: 22.1g
Fiber: 4.1g
Sugar: 9.4g
Protein: 6.8g
Sodium: 87mg

Overnight Fruity Chai Bowl

Serves: 2 individuals
Preparation Time: 10 minutes

Ingredients:
- 2 cups frozen cherries, pitted
- 4 dates, pitted and chopped roughly
- 1 large apple, peeled, cored and chopped
- 1 cup fresh cherries, pitted
- 2 tablespoons chia seeds
- ¼ cup walnuts, chopped

Directions:
1. In a high-powered blender, add frozen cherries and dates and pulse until smooth.
2. In a large-sized bowl, blend together apples, fresh cherries and chia seeds.
3. Add the cherry sauce and stir to blend.
4. Cover and refrigerate to chill overnight.
5. Cover and refrigerate to chill overnight.
6. In the morning, stir the mixture well.
7. Top with walnuts and serve.

Nutritional Information per Serving
Calories: 183
Fat: 6g
Net Carbohydrates: 26.7g
Carbohydrates: 32.7g
Fiber: 6g
Sugar: 25.4g
Protein: 4.5g
Sodium: 1mg

Pumpkin Chia Pudding

Serves: 4 individuals
Preparation Time: 10 minutes

Ingredients:
- 1½ cups unsweetened almond milk
- ½ cup homemade pumpkin puree
- 2 tablespoons organic honey
- 2 tablespoon almond butter
- 1 teaspoon organic vanilla extract
- 1 scoop unflavored protein powder
- 1 teaspoon ground cinnamon
- ¼ teaspoon ground nutmeg
- Pinch of salt
- ¼ cup chia seeds

Directions:
1. Add all ingredients except for chia seeds in a clean blender and pulse until smooth.
2. Transfer the mixture into a bowl.
3. Add chia seeds and stir to blend well.
4. Refrigerate overnight before serving.

Nutritional Information per Serving:
Calories: 168
Fat: 8.8g
Net Carbohydrates: 12.2g
Carbohydrates: 17.1g
Fiber: 4.9g
Sugar: 10.2g
Protein: 10.2g
Sodium: 179mg

Banana Porridge

Serves: 4 individuals
Preparation Time: 10 minutes
Cooking Time: 2 minutes

Ingredients:
- 2 ripe bananas, peeled and mashed
- ¾ cup almond meal
- ¼ cup flaxseed meal
- ½ teaspoon ground ginger
- 1 teaspoon ground cinnamon
- 1/8 teaspoon ground nutmeg
- 1/8 teaspoon ground cloves
- Salt, as needed
- 2 cups unsweetened coconut milk

Directions:
1. In a heavy-bottomed saucepan, add all ingredients and stir to blend.
2. Place the saucepan of banana mixture over medium-low heat and bring to a gentle simmer, stirring continuously.

3. Cook for approximately 2-3 minutes or until desired consistency is achieved, stirring continuously.
4. Serve with your desired topping.

Nutritional Information per Serving:
Calories: 243
Fat: 16g
Net Carbohydrates: 14.2g
Carbohydrates: 20.9g
Fiber: 6.7g
Sugar: 8g
Protein: 2.2g
Sodium: 40mg

Microwave Oatmeal

Serves: 2 individuals
Preparation Time: 10 minutes
Cooking Time: 3 minutes

Ingredients:
- 2/3 cup unsweetened coconut milk
- ½ cup gluten-free quick-cooking oats
- ½ teaspoon ground cinnamon
- ½ teaspoon ground turmeric
- ¼ teaspoon ground ginger

Directions:
1. In a microwave-safe bowl, blend together milk and oats.
2. Microwave on high for approximately 1 minute.
3. Remove from microwave and stir in the spices.
4. Microwave on high for approximately 2 minutes, stirring after every 20 seconds or until desired doneness.
5. Serve immediately.

Nutritional Information per Serving:
Calories: 202
Fat: 12.4g
Net Carbohydrates: 14.3g
Carbohydrates: 16.8g
Fiber: 2.5g
Sugar: 2.2g
Protein: 3.8g
Sodium: 27mg

Pumpkin Quinoa Porridge

Serves: 6 individuals
Preparation Time: 10 minutes
Cooking Time: 22minutes

Ingredients:
- 3½ cups filtered water
- 1¾ cups quinoa, soaked for 15 minutes and rinsed
- 14 ounces unsweetened coconut milk
- 1¾ cups sugar-free pumpkin puree

- 2 teaspoons ground cinnamon
- 1 teaspoon ground ginger
- Pinch of ground cloves
- Pinch of ground nutmeg
- ¼ teaspoon salt
- 3 tablespoons extra-virgin coconut oil
- 3-4 drops liquid stevia
- 1 teaspoon organic vanilla extract

Directions:
1. In a large-sized saucepan, add water and quinoa over high heat.
2. Cover the pan and cook until boiling.
3. Now, adjust the heat to low and simmer for approximately 12-15 minutes or until all the liquid is absorbed.
4. Add remaining ingredients and stir until blended thoroughly.
5. Immediately remove from the heat and serve warm.

Nutritional Information per Serving:
Calories: 370
Fat: 19.2g
Net Carbohydrates: 34.2g
Carbohydrates: 40.2g
Fiber: 6g
Sugar: 4.1g
Protein: 8.7g
Sodium: 124mg

Crepes with Strawberry Sauce

Serves: 2 individuals
Preparation Time: 15 minutes
Cooking Time: 15 minutes

Ingredients:
For Sauce:
- 12 ounces frozen strawberries, thawed and liquid reserved
- 1½ teaspoons tapioca starch
- 1 tablespoon organic honey

For Crepes:
- 2 tablespoons tapioca starch
- 2 tablespoons coconut flour
- ¼ cup unsweetened almond milk
- 2 organic eggs
- Pinch of salt
- Olive oil cooking spray

Directions:
1. For sauce: in a bowl, blend together some reserved strawberry liquid and tapioca starch.
2. Add remaining ingredients and mix well.
3. Transfer the mixture into a saucepan over medium-high heat and cook until boiling, stirring continuously.

4. Cook for approximately 2-3 minutes or until sauce becomes thick, stirring continuously.
5. Remove the pan of sauce from heat and set aside, covered until serving.
6. For crepes: in a clean blender, add all ingredients and pulse until blended thoroughly and smooth.
7. Lightly grease a large-sized non-stick wok with cooking spray and heat over medium-low heat.
8. Add a small-sized amount of mixture and tilt the pan to spread it evenly in the wok.
9. Cook for approximately 1-2 minutes.
10. Carefully change the side and cook for approximately 1-1½ minutes more.
11. Repeat with the remaining mixture.
12. Serve the crepes with the topping of strawberry sauce.

Nutritional Information per Serving:
Calories: 260
Fat: 6.8g
Net Carbohydrates: 00g
Carbohydrates: 43.1g
Fiber: 8.6g
Sugar: 20g
Protein: 7.7g
Sodium: 192mg

Cilantro Pancakes

Serves: 6 individuals
Preparation Time: 15 minutes
Cooking Time: 48 minutes

Ingredients:
- ½ cup tapioca flour
- ½ cup almond flour
- ½ teaspoon red chili powder
- ¼ teaspoon ground turmeric
- Salt and ground black pepper, as needed
- 1 cup full-fat coconut milk
- ½ of red onion, chopped
- 1 (½-inch) piece fresh ginger, grated finely
- 1 Serrano pepper, minced
- ½ cup fresh cilantro, chopped
- Olive oil cooking spray

Directions:
1. In a large-sized bowl, blend together flours and spices.
2. Add coconut milk and mix until blended thoroughly.
3. Fold in the onion, ginger, Serrano pepper and cilantro.
4. Lightly grease a large-sized non-stick wok with cooking spray and heat over medium-low heat.
5. Add about ¼ cup of mixture and tilt the pan to spread it evenly in the wok.
6. Cook for approximately 3-4 minutes from both sides.
7. Repeat with the remaining mixture.
8. Serve warm with your desired topping.

Nutritional Information per Serving:
Calories: 113
Fat: 6.3g
Net Carbohydrates: 10.6g
Carbohydrates: 12g
Fiber: 1.4g
Sugar: 0.5g
Protein: 2.4g
Sodium: 35mg

Pumpkin & Banana Waffles

Serves: 4 individuals
Preparation Time: 15 minutes
Cooking Time: 20 minutes

Ingredients:
- ½ cup almond flour
- ½ cup coconut flour
- 1 teaspoon baking soda
- 1½ teaspoons ground cinnamon
- ¾ teaspoon ground ginger
- ½ teaspoon ground cloves
- ½ teaspoon ground nutmeg
- Salt, as needed
- 2 tablespoons olive oil
- 5 large organic eggs
- ¾ cup unsweetened almond milk
- ½ cup sugar-free pumpkin puree
- 2 medium bananas, peeled and sliced
- Olive oil cooking spray

Directions:
1. In a large-sized bowl, blend together flours, baking soda and spices.
2. In a clean food processor, add the remaining ingredients and pulse until smooth.
3. Add flour mixture and pulse until blended thoroughly.
4. Preheat the waffle iron and then grease it with cooking spray.
5. In the preheated waffle iron, place the required amount of mixture and cook for approximately 4-5 minutes.
6. Repeat with the remaining mixture.
7. Serve warm.

Nutritional Information per Serving
Calories: 312
Fat: 21.5g
Net Carbohydrates: 16.6g
Carbohydrates: 21.9g
Fiber: 5.3g
Sugar: 9.5g
Protein: 12.4g
Sodium: 481mg

Kale Scramble

Serves: 2 individuals
Preparation Time: 10 minutes
Cooking Time: 6 minutes

Ingredients:
- 4 organic eggs
- 2 tablespoons coconut oil
- 2 cups fresh kale, tough ribs removed and chopped
- 1½ teaspoon ground turmeric
- 1 teaspoon garlic powder
- Salt and ground black pepper, as needed

Directions:
1. In a bowl, add eggs and whisk well. Set aside.
2. In a non-stick wok, melt coconut oil over medium heat and cook the kale for approximately 2 minutes.
3. Add eggs and remaining ingredients and cook for approximately 3-4 minutes or until desired doneness, stirring continuously.

Nutritional Information per Serving
Calories: 258
Fat: 22.5g
Net Carbohydrates: 3.2g
Carbohydrates: 4.1g
Fiber: 0.9g
Sugar: 0.8g
Protein: 12g
Sodium: 225mg

Tomato Omelet

Serves: 2 individuals
Preparation Time: 10 minutes
Cooking Time: 6 minutes

Ingredients:
- 4 large organic eggs
- Salt, as needed
- 1 tablespoon olive oil
- 1/8 teaspoon ground turmeric
- ¼ teaspoon brown mustard seeds
- 2 scallions, chopped finely
- ¼ cup tomato, chopped
- Pinch of ground black pepper

Directions:
1. In a bowl, add eggs and salt and whisk well. Set aside.
2. In a cast-iron wok, melt coconut oil over medium-high heat and sauté turmeric and mustard seeds for approximately 30 seconds.
3. Add scallion and sauté for approximately 30 seconds.
4. Add tomato and cook for approximately 1 minute.

5. Add the egg mixture in the wok evenly and cook for approximately 2 minutes.
6. Carefully flip the omelet and cook for approximately 2 minutes more.
7. Transfer the omelet into a plate and cut into 2 wedges.
8. Serve hot with a sprinkling of black pepper.

Nutritional Information per Serving:
Calories: 212
Fat: 17g
Net Carbohydrates: 2.2g
Carbohydrates: 2.9g
Fiber: 0.7g
Sugar: 1.7g
Protein: 13.1g
Sodium: 221mg

Mushroom & Arugula Frittata

Serves: 6 individuals
Preparation Time: 15 minutes
Cooking Time: 25 minutes
Ingredients:
- ½ cup unsweetened coconut milk
- 12 large organic eggs
- Salt, as needed
- 2 tablespoons coconut oil, divided
- 1 small red onion, chopped finely
- 1 cup fresh mushrooms, sliced
- 1 cup fresh arugula, chopped

Directions:
1. Preheat your oven to 375 °F.
2. In a bowl, add coconut milk, eggs and salt and whisk well. Set aside.
3. In an ovenproof wok, heat 1½ tablespoons of oil over medium-high heat and sauté onion for approximately 3 minutes.
4. Add mushrooms and cook for approximately 4-5 minutes.
5. Add arugula and cook for approximately 2-3 minutes.
6. Transfer the vegetable mixture into a bowl.
7. In the same wok, heat the remaining oil over medium-low heat.
8. Add egg mixture and tilt the pan to spread the mixture evenly.
9. Cook for approximately 5 minutes.
10. Spread the vegetable mixture over cooked egg mixture evenly.
11. Immediately, transfer the wok into oven and bake for approximately 5 minutes.
12. Remove the wok from oven and carefully flip the frittata.
13. Bake for approximately 3-4 minutes more.
14. Remove the wok of frittata from oven and set aside for approximately 5 minutes before serving.
15. Cut the frittata into desired-sized wedges and serve.

Nutritional Information per Serving:
Calories: 220
Fat: 17.3g
Net Carbohydrates: 2.5g
Carbohydrates: 2.9g
Fiber: 0.4g
Sugar: 2g
Protein: 13.4g
Sodium: 175mg

Zucchini & Carrot Quiche

Serves: 2 individuals
Preparation Time: 10 minutes
Cooking Time: 40 minutes

Ingredients:
- Olive oil cooking spray
- 5 organic eggs
- Salt and ground black pepper, as needed
- 1 carrot, peeled and grated
- 1 small zucchini, shredded

Directions:
1. Preheat your oven to 350 °F.
2. Lightly grease a small-sized baking dish with cooking spray.
3. In a large-sized bowl, add eggs, salt and black pepper and whisk well.
4. Add carrot and zucchini and stir to blend.
5. Transfer the mixture into the prepared baking dish evenly.
6. Bake for approximately 40 minutes.
7. Remove the baking dish of quiche from oven and set aside for approximately 5 minutes before serving.
8. Cut the quiche into desired-sized wedges and serve.

Nutritional Information per Serving:
Calories: 179
Fat: 11g
Net Carbohydrates: 4.4g
Carbohydrates: 5.8g
Fiber: 1.4g
Sugar: 3.4g
Protein: 14.8g
Sodium: 258mg

Fruity Muffins

Serves: 4 individuals
Preparation Time: 15 minutes
Cooking Time: 25 minutes

Ingredients:
- Olive oil cooking spray
- ½ cup almond meal
- 1 tablespoon linseed meal
- ¼ cup raw sugar
- 2 tablespoons crystallized ginger, chopped finely

- ½ cup buckwheat flour
- ¼ cup brown rice flour
- 2 tablespoons arrowroot flour
- 2 tablespoons organic baking powder
- ½ teaspoon ground ginger
- ½ teaspoon ground cinnamon
- Pinch of salt
- 1 large organic egg
- 7 tablespoons unsweetened almond milk
- ¼ cup extra-virgin olive oil
- 1 teaspoon organic vanilla extract
- 1 small apple, peeled, cored and chopped finely
- 1 cup rhubarb, sliced finely

Directions:
1. Preheat your oven to 350 °F.
2. Grease 8 cups of a large-sized muffin tin with cooking spray.
3. In a large-sized bowl, blend together almond meal, linseed meal, sugar and crystalized ginger.
4. In another bowl, blend together flours, baking powder, spices and salt.
5. Sift the flour mixture into the bowl of almond meal mixture and mix well.
6. In a third bowl, add egg, milk, oil and vanilla and whisk until blended thoroughly.
7. Add egg mixture into flour mixture and mix until blended thoroughly.
8. Fold in apple and rhubarb.
9. Place the mixture into prepared muffin cups evenly.
10. Bake for approximately 20-25 minutes.
11. Remove the muffin tin from oven and place onto a wire rack to cool for approximately 10 minutes.
12. Then invert the muffins onto the wire rack to cool completely before serving.

Nutritional Information per Serving:
Calories: 383
Fat: 21.1g
Net Carbohydrates: 41.6g
Carbohydrates: 47.3g
Fiber: 5.7g
Sugar: 19.9g
Protein: 7.4g
Sodium: 88mg

Carrot & Coconut Muffins

Serves: 6 individuals
Preparation Time: 14 minutes
Cooking Time: 22 minutes

Ingredients:
- 2 cups blanched almond flour
- ½ cup unsweetened coconut shreds
- 1 teaspoon baking soda
- ½ teaspoon ground allspice
- ½ teaspoon ground ginger
- Pinch of ground cloves
- Salt, as needed

- 3 organic eggs
- ½ cup organic honey
- ½ cup coconut oil
- 1 cup carrot, peeled and grated
- 2 tablespoons fresh ginger, peeled and grated
- ¾ cup raisins, soaked in water for 15 minutes and drained

Directions:
1. Preheat your oven to 350 °F.
2. Grease 12 cups of a large-sized muffin tin.
3. In a large-sized bowl, blend together flour, coconut shreds, baking soda, spices and salt.
4. In another bowl, add eggs, honey, and oil and whisk until blended thoroughly.
5. Add egg mixture into flour mixture and mix until blended thoroughly.
6. Fold in carrot, ginger and raisins.
7. Place the mixture into prepared muffin cups evenly.
8. Bake for approximately 20-22 minutes.
9. Remove the muffin tin from oven and place onto a wire rack to cool for approximately 10 minutes.
10. Then invert the muffins onto the wire rack to cool completely before serving.

Nutritional Information per Serving:
Calories: 574
Fat: 41.4g
Net Carbohydrates: 43.1g
Carbohydrates: 48.9g
Fiber: 5.8g
Sugar: 36.7g
Protein: 11.8g
Sodium: 286mg

Veggie Muffins

Serves: 5 individuals
Preparation Time: 15 minutes
Cooking Time: 23 minutes

Ingredients:
- Olive oil cooking spray
- ¾ cup almond meal
- ½ teaspoon baking soda
- ¼ cup whey protein powder
- 2 teaspoons fresh dill, chopped
- Salt, as needed
- 4 large organic eggs
- 1½ tablespoons nutritional yeast
- 2 teaspoons apple cider vinegar
- 3 tablespoons fresh lemon juice
- 2 tablespoons coconut oil, melted
- 1 cup coconut butter, softened
- 1 bunch scallion, chopped
- 2 medium carrots, peeled and grated
- ½ cup fresh parsley, chopped

Directions:

1. Preheat your oven to 350 °F.
2. Grease 10 cups of a large-sized muffin tin with cooking spray.
3. In a large-sized bowl, blend together flour, baking soda, protein powder and salt.
4. In another bowl, add eggs, nutritional yeast, vinegar, lemon juice and oil and whisk until blended thoroughly.
5. Add coconut butter and whisk until mixture becomes smooth.
6. Add egg mixture into flour mixture and mix until blended thoroughly.
7. Fold in scallion, carts and parsley.
8. Place the mixture into prepared muffin cups evenly.
9. Bake for approximately 18-23 minutes.
10. Remove the muffin tin from oven and place onto a wire rack to cool for approximately 10 minutes.
11. Then invert the muffins onto the wire rack and serve warm.

Nutritional Information per Serving:
Calories: 526
Fat: 47g
Net Carbohydrates: 00g
Carbohydrates: 20.1g
Fiber: 11.6g
Sugar: 5.6g
Protein: 13.9g
Sodium: 255mg

Quinoa Bread

Serves: 12 individuals
Preparation Time: 10 minutes
Cooking Time: 1½ hours

Ingredients:

- 1¾ cups uncooked quinoa, soaked overnight and rinsed
- ¼ cup chia seeds, soaked in ½ cup of water overnight
- ½ teaspoon bicarbonate soda
- Salt, as needed
- ¼ cup olive oil
- ½ cup water
- 1 tablespoon fresh lemon juice

Directions:

1. Preheat your oven to 320 °F.
2. Line a loaf pan with parchment paper.
3. In a clean food processor, add all ingredients and pulse for approximately 3 minutes.
4. Place the mixture into the prepared loaf pan evenly.
5. Bake for approximately 1½ hours.
6. Remove the loaf pan from oven and place onto a wire rack to cool for at least 10-15 minutes.
7. Then invert the bread onto the rack to cool completely.

8. Cut the bread loaf into desired-sized slices and serve.

Nutritional Information per Serving:
Calories: 137
Fat: 6.5g
Net Carbohydrates: 14.3g
Carbohydrates: 16.9g
Fiber: 2.6g
Sugar: 0g
Protein: 4g
Sodium: 20mg

Carrot Bread

Serves: 8 individuals
Preparation Time: 15 minutes
Cooking Time: 1 hour

Ingredients:

- 2 cups almond meal
- 1 teaspoon organic baking powder
- 1 tablespoon cumin seeds
- Salt, as needed
- 3 organic eggs
- 2 tablespoons macadamia nut oil
- 1 tablespoon apple cider vinegar
- 3 cups carrot, peeled and grated
- 1 (½-inch) piece fresh ginger, peeled and grated
- ¼ cup sultanas

Directions:

1. Preheat your oven to 350 °F.
2. Line a loaf pan with parchment paper.
3. In a large-sized bowl, blend together almond meal, baking powder, cumin seeds and salt.
4. In another bowl, add eggs, nut oil and vinegar and whisk until blended thoroughly.
5. Add egg mixture into the flour mixture and mix until blended thoroughly.
6. Fold in carrot, ginger and sultanas.
7. Place the mixture into the prepared loaf pan evenly.
8. Bake for approximately 1 hour.
9. Remove the loaf pan from oven and place onto a wire rack to cool for at least 10-15 minutes.
10. Then invert the bread onto the rack to cool completely.
11. Cut the bread loaf into desired-sized slices and serve.

Nutritional Information per Serving:
Calories: 238
Fat: 19.2g
Net Carbohydrates: 7.6g
Carbohydrates: 11.7g
Fiber: 4.1g
Sugar: 3.9g
Protein: 8.6g
Sodium: 73mg

CHAPTER 3:
Sides & Salads
Recipes

Glazed Baby Carrots

Serves: 4 individuals
Preparation Time: 15 minutes
Cooking Time: 15 minutes

Ingredients:
- 2 cups water
- 1 pound baby carrots
- 3 tablespoons maple syrup
- 1 tablespoon coconut oil
- 1 teaspoon ground cinnamon
- Salt, as needed
- 1 tablespoon fresh lemon juice
- 2 tablespoons fresh parsley, chopped
- Ground black pepper, as needed
- 1 tablespoon fresh parsley, minced

Directions:
1. In a medium-sized saucepan, add the water over medium-high heat and cook until boiling.
2. Add the carrots and again cook until boiling.
3. Now, adjust the heat to medium and cook for approximately 6-8 minutes.
4. Drain the carrots well.
5. In a wok, add the maple syrup, coconut oil, lemon juice, salt and black pepper and cook for approximately 5 minutes, stirring continuously.
6. Stir in the parsley and serve warm.

Nutritional Information per Serving:
Calories: 118
Fat: 3.5g
Net Carbohydrates: 18.7g
Carbohydrates: 21.9g
Fiber: 3.2g
Sugar: 14.6g
Protein: 1g
Sodium: 124mg

Spiced Butternut Squash

Serves: 6 individuals
Preparation Time: 10 minutes
Cooking Time: 45 minutes

Ingredients:
- 8 cups butternut squash, peeled, seeded and cubed
- 2 tablespoons almond butter, melted
- ½ teaspoon ground cinnamon
- ½ teaspoon ground cumin
- ¼ teaspoon red pepper flakes
- Salt, as needed

Directions:
1. Preheat your oven to 425 °F.
2. Arrange pieces of foil into 2 baking sheets.
3. In a large-sized bowl, add all the ingredients and toss to combine.
4. Arrange the squash pieces onto the prepared baking sheets in a single layer.
5. Roast for approximately 40-45 minutes.
6. Remove from the oven and serve.

Nutritional Information per Serving:
Calories: 118
Fat: 3.2g
Net Carbohydrates: 18.7g
Carbohydrates: 23.1g
Fiber: 4.4g
Sugar: 4.4g
Protein: 3.1g
Sodium: 35mg

Garlicky Spinach

Serves: 4 individuals
Preparation Time: 10 minutes
Cooking Time: 7 minutes

Ingredients:
- 1 tablespoon olive oil
- 6 garlic cloves, sliced thinly
- 2 (10-ounce) packages fresh spinach
- ½ teaspoon ground turmeric
- ½ teaspoon ground cumin
- 1 tablespoon fresh lemon juice
- Salt and ground black pepper, as needed

Directions:
1. In a large-sized wok, heat oil over medium heat and sauté garlic for approximately 1 minute.
2. Add spinach and spices and cook for approximately 5 minutes.
3. Stir in lemon juice, salt and black pepper and remove from heat.
4. Serve hot.

Nutritional Information per Serving:
Calories: 72
Fat: 4.2g
Net Carbohydrates: 3.7g
Carbohydrates: 7g
Fiber: 3.3g
Sugar: 0.8g
Protein: 4.4g
Sodium: 153mg

Kale with Cranberries & Pine Nuts

Serves: 6 individuals
Preparation Time: 10 minutes
Cooking Time: 14 minutes

Ingredients:

- 2 pounds fresh kale, tough ribs removed and chopped
- 3 tablespoons extra-virgin olive oil
- 1 tablespoon garlic, minced
- ½ cup dried unsweetened cranberries
- Salt and ground black pepper, as needed
- 1/3 cup pine nuts

Directions:

1. In a large-sized saucepan of boiling salted water, cook the kale for approximately 5-7 minutes.
2. In a colander, drain the kale and immediately transfer into an ice bath.
3. Drain the kale and set aside.
4. In a wok, heat the oil over medium heat and sauté the garlic for approximately 1 minute.
5. Add kale, cranberries, salt and black pepper and cook for approximately 4-6 minutes, tossing frequently with tongs.
6. Stir in the pine nuts and serve hot.

Nutritional Information per Serving:
Calories: 196
Fat: 12.2g
Net Carbohydrates: 16.4g
Carbohydrates: 19.3g
Fiber: 2.9g
Sugar: 1.3g
Protein: 5.6g
Sodium: 109mg

Lemony Zoodles

Serves: 8 individuals
Preparation Time: 15 minutes
Cooking Time: 8 minutes

Ingredients:

- 6 zucchinis, spiralized with Blade C
- Salt, as needed
- 3 tablespoons olive oil
- 1 garlic clove, minced
- 2 tablespoons fresh lemon juice
- 2 tablespoons fresh parsley, chopped
- Ground black pepper, as needed

Directions:

1. In a large-sized bowl, add zucchini noodles and salt and toss to combine.
2. Transfer the zucchini noodles into a large-sized colander and set aside or at least 30 minutes to drain.
3. In a pan of boiling water, add zucchini noodles and cook for approximately 1 minute.
4. Drain the zucchini noodles and rinse them under cold water.
5. In a large-sized wok, heat oi over medium-high heat and sauté garlic for approximately 1 minute.

6. Add zucchini noodles and cook for approximately 4-5 minutes.
7. Stir in salt and black pepper and immediately, remove from heat.
8. Serve immediately.

Nutritional Information per Serving:
Calories: 70
Fat: 5.6g
Net Carbohydrates: 3.5g
Carbohydrates: 5.2g
Fiber: 1.7g
Sugar: 2.6g
Protein: 1.9g
Sodium: 35mg

Garlicky Brussels Sprout

Serves: 6 individuals
Preparation Time: 10 minutes
Cooking Time: 15 minutes

Ingredients:

- 1½ pounds fresh Brussels sprouts, trimmed and halved
- 3 garlic cloves, minced
- 2 tablespoons olive oil
- Salt and ground white pepper, as needed

Directions:

1. Preheat your oven to 450 °F.
2. In a large-sized roasting pan, place Brussels sprouts, garlic, oil, salt and black pepper and toss to combine.
3. Then arrange the Brussels sprouts in an even layer.
4. Roast for approximately 10-15 minutes, stirring occasionally.
5. Serve hot.

Nutritional Information per Serving:
Calories: 91
Fat: 5.1g
Net Carbohydrates: 6.5g
Carbohydrates: 10.8g
Fiber: 4.3g
Sugar: 2.5g
Protein: 4g
Sodium: 56mg

Gingered Broccoli

Serves: 2 individuals
Preparation Time: 10 minutes
Cooking Time: 8 minutes

Ingredients:

- 1 tablespoon olive oil
- 2 garlic cloves, minced
- 1 teaspoon fresh ginger, minced
- 2 cups broccoli florets
- 2 tablespoons water
- Salt and ground black pepper, as needed

Directions:

1. In a large-sized wok, heat the oil over medium heat and sauté the garlic and ginger for approximately 1 minute.
2. Add the broccoli and stir fry for 2 minutes.
3. Stir in water, salt, and black pepper and stir fry for 4-5 minutes.
4. Serve hot.

Nutritional Information per Serving:
Calories: 99
Fat: 7.4g
Net Carbohydrates: 5.2g
Carbohydrates: 7.7g
Fiber: 2.5g
Sugar: 1.6g
Protein: 2.8g
Sodium: 109mg

Lemony Mushrooms

Serves: 2 individuals
Preparation Time: 10 minutes
Cooking Time: 15 minutes

Ingredients:

- 2 tablespoons olive oil
- 2-3 tablespoons red onion, minced
- ½ teaspoon garlic, minced
- 12 ounces fresh mushrooms, sliced
- 1 tablespoon fresh parsley
- 2 teaspoons fresh lemon juice
- Salt and ground black pepper, as needed

Directions:

1. In a wok, heat the oil over medium heat and sauté the onion and garlic for 3-4 minutes.
2. Add the mushrooms and cook for 8-10 minutes or until desired doneness.
3. Stir in the parsley, lemon juice, salt and black pepper and remove from the heat.
4. Serve hot.

Nutritional Information per Serving:
Calories: 163
Fat: 14.6g
Net Carbohydrates: 5g
Carbohydrates: 7g
Fiber: 2g
Sugar: 3.5g
Protein: 5.6g
Sodium: 90mg

Bell Peppers with Yellow Squash

Serves: 4 individuals
Preparation Time: 15 minutes
Cooking Time: 10 minutes

Ingredients:

- 1 tablespoon canola oil
- ½ cup onion, sliced
- 1 cup bell pepper, seeded and julienned
- 3 cups yellow squash, sliced
- 1½ teaspoons garlic, minced
- ¼ cup water
- Salt and ground black pepper, as needed

Directions:

1. In a large-sized wok, heat oil over medium-high heat and cook onion, bell peppers and squash for approximately 4-5 minutes.
2. Add garlic and sauté for approximately 1 minute.
3. Stir in remaining ingredients and now, adjust the heat to medium.
4. Cook for approximately 3-4 minutes, stirring occasionally.
5. Serve hot.

Nutritional Information per Serving:
Calories: 61
Fat: 3.8g
Net Carbohydrates: 5.1g
Carbohydrates: 6.8g
Fiber: 1.7g
Sugar: 3.6g
Protein: 1.6g
Sodium: 49mg

Cherry Tomatoes with Green Beans

Serves: 8 individuals
Preparation Time: 15 minutes
Cooking Time: 40 minutes

Ingredients:

- 3-4 garlic cloves, chopped
- 1 teaspoon fresh lemon peel, grated freshly
- 2 teaspoons olive oil
- 1 teaspoon ground cumin
- Salt and ground white pepper, as needed
- 4 cups cherry tomatoes
- 1½ pounds fresh green beans, trimmed

Directions:

1. Preheat your oven to 350 °F.
2. In a large-sized bowl, blend together garlic, lemon peel, oil, cumin, salt and white pepper.
3. Add cherry tomatoes and toss to combine.
4. Transfer the tomato mixture into a roasting pan.
5. Roast for approximately 35-40 minutes, stirring once halfway through.
6. Meanwhile in a pan of boiling water, place steamer basket.

7. Place the green beans in the steamer basket and steam, covered for approximately 7-8 minutes.
8. Drain the green beans well and transfer into a large-sized bowl.
9. Remove the roasting pan from oven.
10. Place the tomatoes into the bowl of green beans stir to blend.
11. Serve immediately.

Nutritional Information per Serving:
Calories: 55
Fat: 1.5g
Net Carbohydrates: 61g
Carbohydrates: 10.1g
Fiber: 4g
Sugar: 3.6g
Protein: 2.5g
Sodium: 30mg

Mango & Bell Pepper Salad
Serves: 6 individuals
Preparation Time: 15 minutes

Ingredients:

For Dressing:
- 1 fresh Serrano pepper, chopped
- 1 tablespoon fresh cilantro, chopped
- 1 teaspoon fresh ginger, chopped
- ¼ cup golden raisins, soaked in boiling water for approximately 30 minutes and drained
- 3 tablespoons extra-virgin olive oil
- 2 tablespoons balsamic vinegar
- Salt, as needed

For Salad:
- 8 cups fresh mixed baby greens
- 2 medium bell peppers, seeded and sliced thinly
- 1 large mango, peeled, pitted and cubed

Directions:
1. For dressing: in a clean blender, add all ingredients and pulse until smooth.
2. Reserve 1 tablespoon of the dressing.
3. In a large-sized bowl, place the greens and remaining dressing and toss to combine.
4. In another bowl, add bell pepper, mango and reserved dressing and toss to coat.
5. Divide the greens and mango mixture in serving bowls.
6. Serve immediately.

Nutritional Information per Serving:
Calories: 131
Fat: 7.4g
Net Carbohydrates: 15.2g
Carbohydrates: 17.4g

Fiber: 2.2g
Sugar: 13.8g
Protein: 1.6g
Sodium: 34mg

Berries & Watermelon Salad
Serves: 8 individuals
Preparation Time: 15 minutes

Ingredients:
- 2½ pound seedless watermelon, cubed
- 2 cups fresh strawberries, hulled and sliced
- 2 cups fresh blueberries
- 1 cup fresh raspberries
- 1 tablespoon fresh ginger root, grated
- 4 tablespoons fresh mint leaves, chopped
- 2 tablespoons organic honey
- ¼ cup fresh lime juice

Directions:
1. In a large-sized salad bowl, add watermelon cubes and remaining ingredients and gently toss to blend.
2. Serve immediately.

Nutritional Information per Serving:
Calories: 101
Fat: 0.6g
Net Carbohydrates: 21.9g
Carbohydrates: 25.3g
Fiber: 3.4g
Sugar: 19.1g
Protein: 1.7g
Sodium: 4mg

Mixed Fruit Salad
Serves: 4 individuals
Preparation Time: 15 minutes

Ingredients:
- 1 fresh pineapple, peeled, cored and chopped
- 2 large mangoes, peeled, pitted and chopped
- 2 large Fuji apples, cored and chopped
- 2 large pears, cored and chopped
- 2 large navel oranges, peeled, seeded and sectioned
- 2 teaspoons fresh ginger, grated finely
- 2 tablespoons organic honey
- ¼ cup fresh lemon juice

Directions:
1. In a large-sized salad bowl, blend together all fruits.
2. In a small-sized bowl, add the remaining ingredients and whisk well.
3. Place honey mixture over fruit mixture and toss to combine.

4. Refrigerate, covered until chilled completely.

Nutritional Information per Serving
Calories: 161
Fat: 0.6g
Net Carbohydrates: 36g
Carbohydrates: 41.6g
Fiber: 5.6g
Sugar: 33.1g
Protein: 1.7g
Sodium: 80mg

Apple, Beet & Carrot Salad
Serves: 6 individuals
Preparation Time: 15 minutes

Ingredients:

For Salad:
- 1¾ cups apple, peeled, cored and grated
- 1¾ cups beetroot, peeled and grated
- 1¾ cups carrots, peeled and grated

For Dressing:
- 1 tablespoon fresh ginger root, grated finely
- 1 tablespoon organic honey
- 3-4 tablespoons fresh lime juice
- 1-3 tablespoons extra-virgin olive oil

Directions:
1. In a large-sized salad bowl, blend together all salad ingredients.
2. In a small-sized bowl, add dressing ingredients and whisk well.
3. Place dressing over salad mixture and toss to combine.
4. Refrigerate before serving.

Nutritional Information per Serving:
Calories: 100
Fat: 2.6g
Net Carbohydrates: 16.7g
Carbohydrates: 20.1g
Fiber: 3.4g
Sugar: 15.2g
Protein: 1.3g
Sodium: 61mg

Collard Greens & Seeds Salad

Serves: 4 individuals
Preparation Time: 15 minutes
Cooking Time: 6 minutes

Ingredients:

- 1½ teaspoons fresh ginger, grated finely
- 2 tablespoons apple cider vinegar
- 3 tablespoons olive oil
- 1 teaspoon sesame oil, toasted
- 3 teaspoons organic honey, divided
- ½ teaspoon red pepper flakes, crushed and divided
- Salt, as needed
- 1 tablespoon water
- 2 tablespoons raw sunflower seeds
- 1 tablespoon raw sesame seeds
- 1 tablespoon raw pumpkin seeds
- 10 ounces fresh collard greens, stems and ribs removed and thinly sliced leaves

Directions:

1. For dressing: in a bowl, add ginger, vinegar, both oils, 1 teaspoon of honey, ¼ teaspoon red pepper flakes and salt and whisk until blended thoroughly. Set aside.
2. In another bowl, add the remaining honey, remaining red pepper flakes and water and mix until blended thoroughly.
3. Heat a medium-sized non-stick wok over medium heat and cook all seeds for approximately 3 minutes, stirring continuously.
4. Stir in the honey mixture and cook for approximately 3 minutes, stirring continuously.
5. Transfer the seeds mixture onto a parchment paper-lined plate and set aside to cool completely.
6. After cooling, break the seeds mixture into small pieces.
7. In a large-sized salad bowl, add the greens, 2 teaspoons of the dressing and a little salt and toss to combine.
8. With your hands, rub the greens for approximately 30 seconds.
9. Add remaining dressing and toss to combine.
10. Serve with a garnishing of seeds pieces.

Nutritional Information per Serving:

Calories: 375
Fat: 14.2g
Net Carbohydrates: 00g
Carbohydrates: 50g
Fiber: 6.5g
Sugar: 18.9g
Protein: 14.2g
Sodium: 109mg

Nutritional Information per Serving

Calories: 184
Fat: 15.6g
Net Carbohydrates: 8.4g
Carbohydrates: 10.5g
Fiber: 2.1g
Sugar: 5g
Protein: 3.6g
Sodium: 389mg

Carrot & Radish Salad

Serves: 4 individuals
Preparation Time: 15 minutes

Ingredients:

- 1 bunch fresh kale, trimmed and sliced thinly
- 1 large garlic clove, minced
- 2 tablespoons coconut aminos
- 2 tablespoons fresh lemon juice
- 3 tablespoon extra-virgin olive oil, divided
- 2 medium carrots, peeled and sliced thinly
- 6 radishes, trimmed and sliced thinly
- 2 tablespoons apple cider vinegar
- 1/3 cup unsweetened coconut flakes, toasted

Directions:

1. In a large-sized bowl, add kale, garlic, coconut aminos, lemon juice and 1 tablespoon of olive oil and toss to combine.
2. With your hands, rub the kale generously.
3. Add in remaining olive oil and toss to combine.
4. Set aside for approximately 15 minutes, stringing occasionally.
5. In another bowl, blend together the carrots, radishes and vinegar.
6. Set aside for approximately 15 minutes, stirring occasionally.
7. Add the carrot mixture in the bowl with kale mixture and toss to blend.
8. Serve with a garnishing of coconut flakes.

Nutritional Information per Serving:

Calories: 168
Fat: 13.7g
Net Carbohydrates: 8.3g
Carbohydrates: 9.4g
Fiber: 1.1g
Sugar: 2.7g
Protein: 0.7g
Sodium: 93mg

Chicken, Jicama & Carrot Salad

Serves: 4 individuals
Preparation Time: 15 minutes

Ingredients:

For Dressing:

- 1 tablespoon fresh ginger, chopped
- 2 tablespoons coconut cream
- 2 tablespoons fresh lime juice
- 1 tablespoon sesame oil
- 1 tablespoon coconut aminos
- 1 tablespoon fish sauce
- 1 teaspoon stevia powder

For Salad:

- 2 cups cooked chicken, chopped
- 1 cup carrot, peeled and chopped
- 2 scallions, chopped
- ½ cup jicama, chopped
- ¼ cup fresh cilantro, chopped
- 1 tablespoon sesame seeds

Directions:
1. For dressing: in a clean blender, add all ingredients and mix until blended thoroughly.
2. In another large salad bowl, blend together salad ingredients.
3. Pour dressing over salad and toss to combine.
4. Serve immediately.

Nutritional Information per Serving:
Calories: 196
Fat: 8.5g
Net Carbohydrates: 5.2g
Carbohydrates: 7.5g
Fiber: 2.3g
Sugar: 2.3g
Protein: 21.7g
Sodium: 19mg

Carbohydrates: 6.2g
Fiber: 2.4g
Sugar: 3.4g
Protein: 27.9g
Sodium: 96mg

Salmon Salad
Serves: 3 individuals
Preparation Time: 10 minutes

Ingredients:
- 1 (14-ounce) can salmon, flaked
- 2 large tomatoes, chopped
- 4 cups fresh baby spinach
- 1 bunch fresh parsley, chopped
- 1 tablespoon fresh lime juice
- Ground black pepper, as needed

Directions:
1. In a large-sized salad bowl, add salmon and remaining ingredients and toss to combine.
2. Serve immediately.

Nutritional Information per Serving:
Calories: 207
Fat: 8.6g
Net Carbohydrates: 3.8g

Black Beans & Mango Salad

Serves: 6 individuals
Preparation Time: 15 minutes

Ingredients:

For Salad:
- 2 (15½-ounce) cans black beans, drained
- 2 mangoes, peeled, pitted and chopped
- ½ cup red onion, chopped
- 2 tablespoons fresh cilantro, chopped

For Dressing:
- 1 (½-inch) pieces fresh ginger, grated
- 2 teaspoons fresh orange zest, grated finely
- 3-4 tablespoons fresh orange juice
- 1 tablespoon apple cider vinegar
- 2 teaspoons extra-virgin olive oil
- ¼ teaspoon red pepper flakes, crushed

Directions:
1. In a large-sized salad bowl, blend together all salad ingredients.
2. In another bowl, add all dressing ingredients and whisk until blended thoroughly.
3. Place dressing over beans mixture and mix until blended thoroughly.
4. Serve immediately.

Nutritional Information per Serving:
Calories: 283
Fat: 2.8g
Net Carbohydrates: 38.6g
Carbohydrates: 53.5g
Fiber: 14.9g
Sugar: 16.4g
Protein: 14.1g
Sodium: 3mg

Lentil & Apple Salad

Serves: 6 individuals
Preparation Time: 15 minutes
Cooking Time: 30 minutes

Ingredients:

For Salad:
- 1 cup French green lentils
- 3 Granny Smith apples, cored and chopped finely
- ½ cup sunflower seeds, toasted
- ½ cup fresh cilantro, chopped

For Dressing:
- 1 teaspoon fresh ginger, grated
- 1 teaspoon organic honey
- ¼ cup fresh lime juice
- ¼ cup extra-virgin olive oil
- Salt and ground black pepper, as needed

Directions:
1. In a large-sized saucepan of water, add lentils over high heat and cook until boiling.
2. Now, adjust the heat to low and simmer, covered for approximately 22-25 minutes.
3. Drain the lentils completely and transfer into a large-sized bowl. Set aside to cool.
4. Add remaining salad ingredients and mix.
5. In another bowl, add all dressing ingredients and whisk until blended thoroughly.
6. Place dressing over lentil mixture and mix until blended thoroughly.
7. Serve immediately.

Nutritional Information per Serving:
Calories: 271
Fat: 10.9g
Net Carbohydrates: 23.8g
Carbohydrates: 36.7g
Fiber: 12.9g
Sugar: 13.3g
Protein: 9.4g
Sodium: 31mg

CHAPTER 4:
Beans & Grains Recipes

Red Kidney Beans Soup

Serves: 4 individuals
Preparation Time: 10 minutes
Cooking Time: 45 minutes

Ingredients:

- 2 (15-ounce) cans red kidney beans, drained
- 1 (14½-ounce) can diced tomatoes
- 1 cup vegetable broth
- 1 (14-ounce) can unsweetened coconut milk
- 2 scallions, chopped
- 2 garlic cloves, minced
- 1 teaspoon fresh ginger, minced
- 1 tablespoon ground cumin
- 1 tablespoon ground ginger
- 1 tablespoon ground turmeric
- Salt, as needed

Directions:

1. In a large-sized Dutch oven, blend together beans and remaining ingredients.
2. Place the pan of beans mixture over medium-high heat and cook until boiling.
3. Now, adjust the heat to low and cook for approximately 30-45 minutes.
4. Serve hot.

Nutritional Information per Serving:

Calories: 373
Fat: 15.5g
Net Carbohydrates: 29.4g
Carbohydrates: 42.9g
Fiber: 13.5g
Sugar: 9.6g
Protein: 15.2g
Sodium: 819mg

Beans & Pasta Soup

Serves: 6 individuals
Preparation Time: 15 minutes
Cooking Time: 35 minutes

Ingredients:

- 2 teaspoons olive oil
- 1 large leek, chopped
- 1 large carrot, peeled and chopped
- 4 garlic cloves, minced
- 1 teaspoon dried rosemary, crushed
- 1 teaspoon red pepper flakes
- 1/8 teaspoon paprika
- 2 large potatoes, peeled and chopped
- 6 cups homemade vegetable broth
- 2 (15-ounce) cans red kidney beans, drained
- 1 (28-ounce) can diced tomatoes
- 1 cup whole-wheat pasta (of your choice)
- Salt and ground black pepper, as needed

Directions:

1. In a large-sized soup pan, heat oil over medium heat and sauté leeks, carrot, garlic, rosemary and spices for approximately 3 minutes.
2. Add broth and potatoes and cook until boiling.
3. Boil for approximately 1-2 minutes.
4. Now, adjust the heat to low and cook, covered for approximately 15 minutes.
5. Stir in beans, tomatoes and pasta and cook for approximately 10 minutes.
6. Stir in salt and black pepper and serve hot.

Nutritional Information per Serving:

Calories: 346
Fat: 4.3g
Net Carbohydrates: 47.8g
Carbohydrates: 60.8g
Fiber: 13g
Sugar: 9.5g
Protein: 17.9g
Sodium: 811mg

Lentils & Veggie Soup

Serves: 6 individuals
Preparation Time: 15 minutes
Cooking Time: 40 minutes

Ingredients:

- 1 tablespoon olive oil
- 4 leeks, chopped
- 1 tablespoon fresh ginger, minced
- 1 tablespoon garlic, minced
- 1 teaspoon ground cumin
- 1 teaspoon ground turmeric
- 1¾ cups tomatoes, chopped
- 6 cups homemade vegetable broth
- ½ cup brown lentils, rinsed
- 2 sweet potatoes, peeled and cubed
- 4 cups fresh kale, tough ribs removed and chopped
- 1 tablespoon fresh thyme, chopped
- Salt and ground black pepper, as needed

Directions:

1. In a large-sized soup pan, heat oil over medium heat and sauté leeks for approximately 3 minutes.
2. Add in the ginger, garlic and spices and sauté for approximately 1 minute.
3. Add tomatoes and cook for 5-6 minutes, crushing with the back of a spoon.
4. Add broth and cook until boiling.
5. Add lentils, sweet potato, kale, and thyme and again cook until boiling.
6. Now adjust the heat to low and simmer, covered for approximately 25-30 minutes or until desired doneness.
7. Stir in salt and black pepper and serve hot.

Nutritional Information per Serving:

Calories: 245
Fat: 4.3g
Net Carbohydrates: 30.4g
Carbohydrates: 40.2g
Fiber: 9.8g
Sugar: 6.1g
Protein: 12.8g
Sodium: 832mg

Chickpeas & Squash Stew

Serves: 4 individuals
Preparation Time: 15 minutes
Cooking Time: 1¼ hours

Ingredients:

- 2 tablespoons avocado oil
- 1 large white onion, chopped
- 4 garlic cloves, minced
- 1 tablespoon fresh ginger, minced
- ½ tablespoon cayenne powder
- 4 large plum tomatoes, seeded and chopped finely
- 1 pound butternut squash, peeled, seeded and chopped
- 2 cups water
- 1½ cups cooked chickpeas
- 2 tablespoons fresh lime juice
- Salt and ground black pepper, as needed
- 2 tablespoons fresh parsley, chopped

Directions:

1. In a soup pan, heat the avocado oil over medium heat and sauté the onion for approximately 4-6 minutes.
2. Add the garlic and cayenne powder and sauté for approximately 1 minute.
3. Add the tomatoes and cook for approximately 2-3 minutes.
4. Add the squash and water and cook until boiling.
5. Now, adjust the heat to low and simmer, covered for approximately 50 minutes.
6. Add the chickpeas and cook for approximately 10 minutes.
7. Stir in lime juice, salt and black pepper and remove from heat.
8. Serve hot with the garnishing of parsley.

Nutritional Information per Serving:

Calories: 223
Fat: 2.6g
Net Carbohydrates: 36.3g
Carbohydrates: 46.1g
Fiber: 9.8g
Sugar: 9g
Protein: 8g
Sodium: 109mg

Black Beans Stew

Serves: 4 individuals
Preparation Time: 10 minutes
Cooking Time: 30 minutes

Ingredients:
- 1 tablespoon olive oil
- 2 small onions, chopped
- 1 small carrot, peeled and chopped
- 5 garlic cloves, chopped finely
- 1 teaspoon of dried oregano
- 1 teaspoon ground cumin
- ½ teaspoon ground ginger
- Salt and ground black pepper, as needed
- 1 (14-ounce) can diced tomatoes
- 2 (13½-ounce) cans black beans, drained
- ½ cup vegetable broth

Directions:
1. Heat the olive oil in a pan over medium heat and cook the onion and carrot for approximately 5-7 minutes, stirring frequently.
2. Add garlic, oregano, spices, salt and black pepper and cook for approximately 1 minute.
3. Add the tomatoes and cook for approximately 1-2 minutes.
4. Add in the beans and broth and cook until boiling.
5. Now, adjust the heat to medium-low and simmer, covered for approximately 15 minutes.
6. Serve hot.

Nutritional Information per Serving:
Calories: 334
Fat: 5.1g
Net Carbohydrates: 36.5g
Carbohydrates: 55.7g
Fiber: 19.2g
Sugar: 4.9g
Protein: 19.3g
Sodium: 153mg

Lentil & Potato Stew

Serves: 4 individuals
Preparation Time: 15 minutes
Cooking Time: 55 minutes

Ingredients:
- 1 cup dry lentils, drained
- 1 cup potato, peeled and chopped
- ½ cup celery, chopped
- ½ cup carrot, peeled and chopped
- ½ cup onion, chopped
- 1 garlic clove, minced
- 1 (14½-ounce) can peeled Italian tomatoes, chopped
- 1 tablespoon dried basil, crushed
- 1 tablespoon dried parsley, crushed
- Salt and ground black pepper, as needed
- 3½ cups chicken bones broth

Directions:
1. In a large-sized Dutch oven, add all ingredients and stir to blend.
2. Place the Dutch oven over high heat and cook until boiling.
3. Now, adjust the heat to low and simmer, covered for approximately 45-50 minutes, stirring occasionally.
4. Serve hot.

Nutritional Information per Serving:
Calories: 269
Fat: 2.1g
Net Carbohydrates: 26.5g
Carbohydrates: 44.3g
Fiber: 17.8g
Sugar: 6.2g
Protein: 19g
Sodium: 677mg

Spicy Black Beans with Tomatoes

Serves: 6 individuals
Preparation Time: 150 minutes
Cooking Time: 1½ hours

Ingredients:

- 4 cups water
- 1½ cups dried black beans, soaked for 8 hours and drained
- ½ teaspoon ground turmeric
- 3 tablespoons olive oil
- 1 teaspoon cumin seeds
- 1 teaspoon black mustard seeds
- 1 small onion, chopped finely
- 2 green chilies, chopped
- 1 (1-inch) piece fresh ginger, minced
- 1 garlic clove, minced
- 1 tablespoon dried curry leaves
- 1 tablespoon dried fenugreek leaves
- 1½ tablespoons ground coriander
- 1 teaspoon garam masala powder
- 1 teaspoon ground cumin
- ½ teaspoon mustard powder
- ½ teaspoon ground turmeric
- ½ teaspoon cayenne powder
- Salt, as needed
- 2 medium tomatoes, chopped finely
- ½ cup fresh cilantro, chopped

Directions:

1. In a large-sized saucepan, add water, black beans and turmeric over high heat and cook until boiling.
2. Now, adjust the heat to low and cook, covered for approximately 1 hour.
3. Meanwhile, in a medium-sized wok, heat oil over medium heat and sauté cumin seeds and mustard seeds for approximately 1 minute.
4. Add onion and sauté for approximately 4-5 minutes.
5. Add green chilies, ginger and garlic and sauté for approximately 1-2 minutes.
6. Add dried leaves and spices and sauté for approximately 1 minute.
7. Stir in tomatoes and cook for approximately 10 minutes, stirring occasionally.
8. Transfer the tomato mixture into the pan with black beans and stir to blend.
9. Now, adjust the heat to medium-low and cook for approximately 15-20 minutes.
10. Stir in cilantro and simmer for approximately 5 minutes.
11. Serve hot.

Nutritional Information per Serving:

Calories: 214
Fat: 8g
Net Carbohydrates: 21.1g
Carbohydrates: 28.6g
Fiber: 7.5g
Sugar: 1.7g
Protein: 9.2g
Sodium: 33mg

Chickpeas with Potatoes

Serves: 6 individuals
Preparation Time: 15 minutes
Cooking Time: 40 minutes

Ingredients:

- 2 tablespoons olive oil
- 1 onion, chopped
- 1 teaspoon fresh ginger, minced
- 2 garlic cloves, minced
- 1 tablespoon hot curry powder
- 1 teaspoon ground cumin
- ¼ teaspoon ground turmeric
- 2 (15-ounce) cans chickpeas, drained
- 2 large potatoes, scrubbed and cubed
- 2 (15-ounce) cans diced tomatoes with liquid
- 2 cups homemade vegetable broth
- Salt and ground black pepper, as needed
- ¼ cup fresh cilantro, chopped

Directions:

1. In a large-sized saucepan, heat oil over medium heat and cook onion for approximately 4-5 minutes.
2. Add ginger, garlic, curry powder and spices and sauté for approximately 1 minute.
3. Add potatoes and cook for approximately 3-4 minutes.
4. Add in chickpeas and remaining ingredients except for cilantro and cook until boiling.
5. Now, adjust the heat to medium-low and cook, covered for approximately 15-25 minutes or until desired doneness.
6. Serve hot with the garnishing of cilantro.

Nutritional Information per Serving:

Calories: 344
Fat: 7.3g
Net Carbohydrates: 48.3g
Carbohydrates: 59.7g
Fiber: 11.4g
Sugar: 6.2g
Protein: 12.3g
Sodium: 722mg

Kidney Beans Curry

Serves: 6 individuals
Preparation Time: 15 minutes
Cooking Time: 25 minutes

Ingredients:
- 4 tablespoons olive oil
- 1 medium onion, chopped finely
- 2 garlic cloves, minced
- 2 tablespoons fresh ginger, minced
- 1 teaspoon ground coriander
- 1 teaspoon ground cumin
- ½ teaspoon ground turmeric
- ¼ teaspoon cayenne pepper
- Salt and ground black pepper, as needed
- 2 large plum tomatoes, chopped finely
- 3 cups cooked red kidney beans
- 2 cups water
- ¼ cup fresh cilantro, chopped

Directions:
1. In a large-sized saucepan, heat oil over medium heat and sauté the onion, garlic, and ginger for approximately 3-4 minutes.
2. Stir in spices cook for approximately 1 minute.
3. Add in tomatoes, kidney beans and water and stir to blend.
4. Now adjust the heat to high and cook until boiling.
5. Now, adjust the heat to medium and cook for approximately 10-15 minutes.
6. Serve hot with the garnishing of parsley.

Nutritional Information per Serving:
Calories: 213
Fat: 10.2g
Net Carbohydrates: 17g
Carbohydrates: 24g
Fiber: 7g
Sugar: 3g
Protein: 8.5g
Sodium: 109mg

Black Beans & Veggie Chili

Serves: 6 individuals
Preparation Time: 15 minutes
Cooking Time: 1 hour

Ingredients:
For Spice Mixture:
- 1 teaspoon ground cinnamon
- ½ teaspoon ground nutmeg
- 1/8 teaspoon ground cloves
- 1 tablespoon red chili powder
- ¼ teaspoon cayenne powder
- Salt, as needed

For Chili:
- 2 teaspoons olive oil
- 1 medium onion, chopped
- 1 jalapeño pepper, seeded and chopped
- 2 tablespoons fresh ginger, minced
- 2 large garlic cloves, minced
- 4 large Portobello mushrooms, stemmed and cubed
- 2 medium carrots, peeled and cubed
- 1 (15-ounce) can black beans, drained
- 2 cups frozen corn
- 1 (28-ounce) can fire roasted tomatoes
- 1 (15-ounce) can sugar-free pumpkin puree
- 2 cups homemade vegetable broth

Directions:
1. For spice mixture: in a bowl, blend together all ingredients. Set aside.
2. In a large-sized, heavy-bottomed saucepan, heat oil over medium heat and cook onion, jalapeño pepper, ginger and garlic for approximately 3-4 minutes.
3. Add mushrooms and carrots and cook for approximately 6 minutes, stirring occasionally.
4. Stir in spice mixture and remaining ingredients and cook until boiling.
5. Now, adjust the heat to medium-low and cook, covered for approximately 40-45 minutes.
6. Serve hot.

Nutritional Information per Serving:
Calories: 244
Fat: 3.9g
Net Carbohydrates: 00g
Carbohydrates: 44.6g
Fiber: 13.3g
Sugar: 10g
Protein: 12.7g
Sodium: 329mg

Three Beans Chili

Serves: 4 individuals
Preparation Time: 15 minutes
Cooking Time: 1 hour 5 minutes

Ingredients:
For spice Mixture:

- 1 teaspoon dried oregano, crushed
- 1 tablespoon red chili powder
- 1 tablespoon red pepper flakes, crushed
- 2 teaspoons ground cumin
- 1 teaspoon ground turmeric
- 1 teaspoon onion powder
- 1 teaspoon garlic powder
- 1 teaspoon paprika
- Salt and ground black pepper, as needed

For Chili:
- 2 tablespoons olive oil
- 1 red bell pepper, seeded and chopped

- 1 green bell pepper, seeded and chopped
- 3 large celery stalks, chopped
- 1 scallion, chopped
- 3 garlic cloves, minced
- 1 (28-ounce) can diced tomatoes
- 4 cups water
- 1 (16-ounce) can kidney beans, drained
- 1 (16-ounce) can cannellini beans, drained
- 1 (8-ounce) can black beans, drained
- 1 jalapeño pepper, seeded and chopped

Directions:
1. For spice mixture: in a small-sized bowl, blend together all ingredients. Set aside.
2. In a large-sized saucepan, heat oil over medium heat and cook bell peppers, celery, scallion and garlic for approximately 8-10 minutes.
3. Add spice mixture, tomatoes and water and cook until boiling.
4. Now, adjust the heat to low and cook for approximately 20 minutes.
5. Stir in beans and jalapeño pepper and simmer for approximately 30 minutes.
6. Serve hot.

Nutritional Information per Serving
Calories: 342
Fat: 6.1g
Net Carbohydrates: 34.7g
Carbohydrates: 56g
Fiber: 21.3g
Sugar: 6g
Protein: 20.3g
Sodium: 79mg

Chickpeas Chili
Serves: 4 individuals
Preparation Time: 15 minutes
Cooking Time: 30 minutes

Ingredients:
- 2 teaspoons olive oil
- 1 cup onion, chopped
- ½ cup carrot, peeled and chopped
- ¾ cup celery, chopped
- 1 teaspoon garlic, minced
- 2 teaspoons ground cumin
- 1 teaspoon ground ginger
- ½ teaspoon ground turmeric
- 1/8 teaspoon ground cinnamon
- 2 teaspoons paprika
- 1/8 teaspoon red chili powder
- Salt and ground black pepper, as needed
- 2 (15½-ounce) cans chickpeas, drained
- 1 (14½-ounce) can diced tomatoes
- 2 tablespoons sugar-free tomato paste
- 1½ cups water

- 1 tablespoon fresh lemon juice
- 2 tablespoons fresh cilantro, chopped

Directions:
1. In a large-sized saucepan, heat oil over medium heat and cook onion, carrot, celery and garlic for approximately 5 minutes.
2. Add spices and sauté for approximately 1 minute.
3. Add chickpeas, tomatoes, tomato paste and water and cook until boiling.
4. Now, adjust the heat to low and simmer, covered for approximately 20 minutes.
5. Stir in lemon juice and cilantro and serve hot.

Nutritional Information per Serving:
Calories: 339
Fat: 5.6g
Net Carbohydrates: 48.5g
Carbohydrates: 61.8g
Fiber: 13.2g
Sugar: 6.1g
Protein: 13.2g
Sodium: 748mg

Lentil Chili
Serves: 8 individuals
Preparation Time: 15 minutes
Cooking Time: 2 hours 10 minutes

Ingredients:
- 2 teaspoons olive oil
- 1 large onion, chopped
- 3 medium carrots, peeled and chopped
- 4 celery stalks, chopped
- 2 garlic cloves, minced
- 2 tablespoons tomato paste
- 1½ tablespoons ground coriander
- 1½ tablespoons ground cumin
- 1½ teaspoons ground turmeric
- 1 teaspoon chipotle chili powder
- Salt and ground black pepper, as needed
- 1 pound lentils, rinsed
- 8 cups homemade vegetable broth
- 1 cup fresh spinach, chopped
- ¼ cup fresh cilantro, chopped

Directions:
1. In a large-sized saucepan, heat oil over medium heat and cook onion, carrot and celery and sauté for approximately 3-5 minutes.
2. Add garlic, tomato paste and spices and sauté for approximately 1 minute.
3. Add lentils and broth and cook until boiling.
4. Now, adjust the heat to low and simmer for approximately 2 hours.
5. Stir in spinach and cook for approximately 3-4 minutes.

6. Serve hot with the garnishing of cilantro.

Nutritional Information per Serving:
Calories: 296
Fat: 5.3g
Net Carbohydrates: 27.7g
Carbohydrates: 47.3g
Fiber: 19.6g
Sugar: 9g
Protein: 17.1g
Sodium: 93mg

Mixed Grains Chili

Serves: 12 individuals
Preparation Time: 15 minutes
Cooking Time: 55 minutes

Ingredients:
- 2 tablespoons olive oil
- 2 shallots, chopped
- 1 large yellow onion, chopped
- 1 tablespoon fresh ginger, grated finely
- 8 garlic cloves, minced
- 1 teaspoon ground cumin
- 3 tablespoons red chili powder
- Salt and ground black pepper, as needed
- 1 (28-ounce) can crushed tomatoes
- 1 canned chipotle pepper, minced
- 1 Serrano pepper, seeded and chopped finely
- 2/3 cup bulgur wheat
- 2/3 cup pearl barley
- 2¼ cups mixed lentils (green, black, brown), rinsed
- 1½ cups canned chickpeas
- 3 scallions, chopped

Directions:
1. In a large-sized saucepan heat oil over medium heat and cook shallot and onion for approximately 3-4 minutes.
2. Add ginger, garlic, cumin and chili powder and sauté for approximately 1 minute.
3. Add the tomatoes, both peppers and broth and stir to blend.
4. Stir in the bulgur, barley, lentils and chickpeas and cook until boiling.
5. Now, adjust the heat to low and cook for approximately 35-45 minutes or until desired thickness of the chili.
6. Serve hot with the topping of scallion.

Nutritional Information per Serving
Calories: 337
Fat: 4.6g
Net Carbohydrates: 38.8g
Carbohydrates: 59.7g
Fiber: 20.9g
Sugar: 4.3g

Protein: 17g
Sodium: 143mg

Black-Eyed Peas Curry

Serves: 3 individuals
Preparation Time: 15 minutes
Cooking Time: 15 minutes

Ingredients:
- 1 teaspoon olive oil
- 1 onion, chopped
- 2 teaspoons fresh ginger, minced
- 3 garlic cloves, minced
- 2 green chilies, split in half
- 1 tablespoon fresh thyme, chopped
- 2 teaspoons curry powder
- ½ teaspoon ground cumin
- 1 (16-ounce) can black-eyed peas, drained and rinsed
- ¾ cup water
- ¾ cup coconut milk
- 1 teaspoon applesauce
- 1 tablespoon fresh lime juice
- Salt and ground black pepper, as needed
- 2 tablespoons fresh parsley, chopped

Directions:
1. In a large-sized Dutch oven, heat oil over medium heat and sauté the onion for 4-5 minutes.
2. Add the ginger, garlic, green chili, thyme, curry powder, and cumin and sauté for about 1 minute.
3. Add the black-eyed peas, water, coconut milk, and applesauce and bring to a boil.
4. Cover and cook for 5 minutes.
5. Stir in the lime juice, salt, and black pepper and cook or about 1 minute.
6. serve hot with a garnish of parsley.

Nutritional Information per Serving:
Calories: 297
Fat: 17.6g
Net Carbohydrates: 22.2g
Carbohydrates: 30.4g
Fiber: 8.2g
Sugar: 3.9g
Protein: 9.9g
Sodium: 126mg

Spicy Lentils Curry

Serves: 8 individuals
Preparation Time: 10 minutes
Cooking Time: 45 minutes

Ingredients:

- 2 cups red lentils, rinsed
- 1 tablespoon olive oil
- 1 large onion, chopped
- 1 teaspoon fresh ginger, minced
- 1 teaspoon garlic, minced
- 2 tablespoons curry paste
- 1 tablespoon curry powder
- 1 teaspoon ground cumin
- 1 teaspoon ground turmeric
- 1 teaspoon red chili powder
- Salt and ground black pepper, as needed
- 1 (14¼-ounce) can tomato puree

Directions:

1. In a large-sized saucepan of water, add lentils over high heat and cook until boiling.
2. Now, adjust the heat to medium-low and simmer, covered for approximately 15-20 minutes.
3. Drain the lentils well.
4. In a large-sized wok, heat oil over medium heat and cook the onion for approximately 10 minutes.
5. Meanwhile, in a bowl, blend together ginger, garlic, spices, salt and black pepper.
6. Add spice mixture into the wok with onions and stir to blend.
7. Cook for approximately 1-2 minutes, stirring continuously.
8. Stir in tomato puree and cook for approximately 1 minute.
9. Transfer the mixture into the pan with the lentils and stir to blend.
10. Serve hot.

Nutritional Information per Serving:

Calories: 192
Fat: 2.6g
Net Carbohydrates: 21.2g
Carbohydrates: 32.5g
Fiber: 11.3g
Sugar: 6.6g
Protein: 12.1g
Sodium: 572mg

Lentils with Spinach

Serves: 4 individuals
Preparation Time: 15 minutes
Cooking Time: 35 minutes

Ingredients:

- 3½ cups water
- 1½ cups red lentils, soaked for 20 minutes and drained
- ½ teaspoon red chili powder
- ½ teaspoon ground turmeric
- Salt, as needed
- 1 pound fresh spinach, chopped
- 2 tablespoons coconut oil
- 1 onion, chopped
- 1 teaspoon mustard seeds
- 1 teaspoon ground cumin
- ½ cup unsweetened coconut milk
- 1 teaspoon garam masala powder

Directions:

1. In a large-sized saucepan, add water, lentils, red chili powder, turmeric and salt over high heat and cook until boiling.
2. Now, adjust the heat to low and simmer, covered for approximately 15 minutes.
3. Stir in spinach and simmer for approximately 5 minutes.
4. In a frying pan, melt coconut oil over medium heat and cook onion, mustard seeds and cumin and sauté for approximately 4-5 minutes.
5. Transfer the onion mixture into the pan with the lentils and stir to blend.
6. Stir in coconut milk and garam masala and simmer for approximately 3-5 minutes.
7. Serve hot.

Nutritional Information per Serving:

Calories: 362
Fat: 13.4g
Net Carbohydrates: 26.6g
Carbohydrates: 44.9g
Fiber: 18.3g
Sugar: 5.5g
Protein: 21g
Sodium: 693mg

Beans & Quinoa with Veggies

Serves: 6 individuals
Preparation Time: 15 minutes
Cooking Time: 35 minutes

Ingredients:

- 2 cups water
- 1 cup dry quinoa
- 2 tablespoons coconut oil
- 1 medium onion, chopped
- 4 garlic cloves, chopped finely
- 2 tablespoons curry powder
- ½ teaspoon ground turmeric
- ½ teaspoon cayenne powder
- Salt, as needed
- 2 cups broccoli, chopped
- 1 cup fresh kale, trimmed and chopped
- 1 cup green peas, shelled
- 1 red bell pepper, seeded and chopped
- 2 cups canned kidney beans, drained
- 2 tablespoons fresh lime juice

Directions:

1. In a large-sized saucepan, add water over high heat and cook until boiling.
2. Add quinoa and immediately adjust the heat to low.
3. Simmer for approximately 10-15 minutes or until all the liquid is absorbed.
4. In a large-sized wok, melt coconut oil over medium heat and cook onion, garlic, curry powder, turmeric and salt for approximately 4-5 minutes.
5. Add the vegetables and cook for approximately 5-6 minutes.
6. Stir in quinoa and beans and cook for approximately 3-4 minutes.
7. Drizzle with lime juice and serve.

Nutritional Information per Serving:

Calories: 276
Fat: 7.2g
Net Carbohydrates: 33.2g
Carbohydrates: 43.5g
Fiber: 10.3g
Sugar: 5.4g
Protein: 11.8g
Sodium: 270mg

Quinoa in Tomato Sauce

Serves: 4 individuals
Preparation Time: 10 minutes
Cooking Time: 40 minutes

Ingredients:

- 2 tablespoons olive oil
- 1 cup quinoa
- 1 green bell pepper, seeded and chopped
- 1 medium onion, chopped finely
- 1 tablespoon fresh ginger, minced
- 3 garlic cloves, minced
- 2½ cups water
- 1 (8-ounce) can sugar-free tomato sauce
- 1 teaspoon red chili powder
- ¼ teaspoon ground cumin
- ¼ teaspoon garlic powder

Directions:

1. In a large-sized saucepan, heat oil over medium-high heat and stir fry quinoa, onion, bell pepper, ginger and garlic for approximately 5 minutes, stirring continuously.
2. Add in water and remaining ingredients and cook until boiling.
3. Now, adjust the heat to medium-low and cook, covered for approximately 30 minutes, stirring occasionally.
4. Serve hot.

Nutritional Information per Serving:

Calories: 262
Fat: 10g
Net Carbohydrates: 32.1g
Carbohydrates: 37.4g
Fiber: 5.3g
Sugar: 5.2g
Protein: 7.7g
Sodium: 328mg

Brown Rice & Mushroom Bake

Serves: 2 individuals
Preparation Time: 15 minutes
Cooking Time: 1 hour

Ingredients:

- 1 teaspoon extra-virgin olive oil
- 1 red onion, sliced thinly
- 1½ teaspoons ground turmeric
- 9 ounces brown mushrooms, sliced
- 1 teaspoon raisins
- ½ cup brown rice, rinsed
- 1¼ cups homemade vegetable broth
- ¼ cup fresh cilantro, chopped
- ½ tablespoons pine nuts, toasted
- 1 tablespoon fresh lemon juice
- Salt and ground black pepper, as needed

Directions:

1. Preheat your oven to 400 °F.
2. In an ovenproof saucepan, heat oil over medium heat and cook onion and turmeric for approximately 3 minutes.
3. Add mushrooms and stir fry for approximately 2 minutes.
4. Stir in raisins, rice and broth and transfer into oven.
5. Bake for approximately 45-55 minutes or until desired doneness.
6. Remove the pan of rice mixture from heat and stir in remaining ingredients.
7. Serve hot.

Nutritional Information per Serving:

Calories: 201
Fat: 5g
Net Carbohydrates: 30.2g
Carbohydrates: 33.7g
Fiber: 3.5g
Sugar: 10.8g
Protein: 6.7g
Sodium: 384mg

CHAPTER 5:
Poultry Recipes

Chicken & Tomato Soup

Serves: 4 individuals
Preparation Time: 15 minutes
Cooking Time: 23 minutes

Ingredients:
- 4 cups chicken bones broth
- 2 large tomatoes, peeled, seeded and chopped
- 1 jalapeño pepper, seeded and minced
- 1 garlic clove, minced
- 1 teaspoon fresh ginger, minced
- ½ teaspoon ground cumin
- 2 cups cooked chicken, shredded
- 3 scallions, finely chopped
- Salt, as needed
- ¼ cup fresh cilantro, chopped
- 2 tablespoons fresh lime juice

Directions:
1. In a soup pan, add broth over medium heat and cook until boiling.
2. Add the tomatoes, jalapeño pepper, garlic, ginger and cumin and simmer for approximately 15 minutes.
3. Add the chicken, scallion and salt and stir to blend.
4. Now adjust the heat to low and simmer for approximately 1-2 minutes.
5. Stir in the cilantro and lime juice and remove the soup pan from heat.
6. Serve immediately.

Nutritional Information per Serving:
Calories: 166
Fat: 2.4g
Net Carbohydrates: 3.8g
Carbohydrates: 5.4g
Fiber: 1.6g
Sugar: 2.8g
Protein: 30.5g
Sodium: 54mg

Chicken & Veggie Soup

Serves: 8 individuals
Preparation Time: 20 minutes
Cooking Time: 40 minutes

Ingredients:
- 1½ tablespoons olive oil
- 1 large onion, chopped
- 2 large potatoes, peeled and chopped
- 4 parsnips, peeled and chopped
- 2 zucchinis, chopped
- 1 cup fresh green peas, shelled
- 4 (6-ounce) boneless, skinless chicken breasts

- 2 teaspoons ground cumin
- 1 tablespoon ground turmeric
- 4 cups chicken bones broth
- 6 cups water
- ½ cup fresh cilantro, chopped

Directions:
1. In a large-sized soup pan, heat oil over medium heat and cook onion for approximately 3-5 minutes stirring continuously.
2. Stir in vegetables and cook for approximately 5 minutes.
3. Stir in remaining ingredients and cook until boiling.
4. Now, adjust the heat to medium-low and cook, covered for approximately 10-15 minutes
5. With a slotted spoon, remove the chicken breasts from soup and place into a bowl.
6. With two forks, shred the chicken breasts.
7. Return the shredded chicken into the soup and simmer for approximately 10 minutes.
8. Serve hot with the garnishing of cilantro.

Nutritional Information per Serving:
Calories: 342
Fat: 9.6g
Net Carbohydrates: 24.2g
Carbohydrates: 31.2g
Fiber: 7g
Sugar: 6.4g
Protein: 33.3g
Sodium: 145mg

Turkey & Veggies Soup

Serves: 8 individuals
Preparation Time: 15 minutes
Cooking Time: 20 minutes

Ingredients:
- 8 cups chicken bones broth
- 2-3 cups broccoli, chopped
- 8 ounces fresh mushrooms, sliced
- 6 scallions, chopped
- 1 (1-inch) piece fresh ginger root, minced
- 4 garlic cloves, minced
- 1½ pounds cooked turkey meat, thinly sliced
- ½ teaspoon ground cumin
- ½ teaspoon ground turmeric
- ½ teaspoon red pepper flakes, crushed
- 2 tablespoons fresh lime juice

Directions:
1. In a large-sized soup pan, add the broth over high heat and cook until boiling.
2. Stir in broccoli pieces and cook for approximately 1-2 minutes.
3. Stir in mushroom, scallions, ginger and garlic and cook for approximately 7-8 minutes.

4. Stir in turkey meat, spices and lime juice and adjust the heat to low.
5. Simmer for approximately 3-5 minutes.
6. Serve hot.

Nutritional Information per Serving
Calories: 203
Fat: 5.8g
Net Carbohydrates: 3.5g
Carbohydrates: 4.6g
Fiber: 1.1g
Sugar: 1.8g
Protein: 31.6g
Sodium: 533mg

Ground Turkey & Cabbage Soup

Serves: 8 individuals
Preparation Time: 15 minutes
Cooking Time: 45 minutes

Ingredients:
- 1 tablespoon olive oil
- 1 large onion, chopped
- 1 pound lean ground turkey
- 2 garlic cloves, minced
- 1 tablespoon fresh ginger, minced
- 1 teaspoon salt
- ½ teaspoon ground black pepper
- 6 cups cabbage, shredded
- 2½ cups tomatoes, chopped finely
- ½ teaspoon dried thyme
- ½ teaspoon dried oregano
- 1 bay leaf
- ½ teaspoon paprika
- ½ teaspoon ground cumin
- ½ teaspoon ground cinnamon
- 6 cups chicken bones broth

Directions:
1. In a large-sized soup pan, heat the oil over medium-high heat and sauté the onion for approximately 3-5 minutes.
2. Add the ground turkey, garlic, ginger, salt and black pepper and stir to blend.
3. Now, adjust the heat to medium-high and cook for approximately 7-8 minutes.
4. Add the cabbage, tomatoes, herbs, bay leaf, spices and broth and cook until boiling.
5. Now, adjust the heat to low and simmer for approximately 25 minutes.
6. Season with more salt and black pepper and serve hot.

Nutritional Information per Serving:
Calories: 210

Fat: 6.7g
Net Carbohydrates: 7.4g
Carbohydrates: 10.8g
Fiber: 3.4g
Sugar: 5.9g
Protein: 26.6g
Sodium: 809mg

Chicken & Tomato Stew

Serves: 8 individuals
Preparation Time: 15 minutes
Cooking Time: 30 minutes

Ingredients:
- 2 tablespoons olive oil
- 1 onion, chopped
- ½ tablespoon fresh ginger, grated finely
- 1 tablespoon fresh garlic, minced
- 1 teaspoon ground turmeric
- 1 teaspoon ground cumin
- 1 teaspoon ground coriander
- 1 teaspoon paprika
- 1 teaspoon cayenne powder
- 6 (6-ounce) skinless, boneless chicken thighs, cut into 1-inch pieces
- 3 Roma tomatoes, chopped
- 1 (14-ounce) can unsweetened coconut milk
- Salt and ground black pepper, as needed
- 1/3 cup fresh cilantro, chopped

Directions:
1. In a large-sized saucepan, heat oil over medium heat and cook onion for approximately 8-10 minutes.
2. Add ginger, garlic and spices and sauté for approximately 1 minute.
3. Add chicken and cook for approximately 4-5 minutes.
4. Add tomatoes, coconut milk, salt and black pepper and brig to gentle simmer.
5. Now, adjust the heat to low and simmer, covered for approximately 10-15 minutes or until desired doneness.
6. Stir in cilantro and serve hot.

Nutritional Information per Serving:
Calories: 395
Fat: 29.8g
Net Carbohydrates: 4.3g
Carbohydrates: 5.5g
Fiber: 1.2g
Sugar: 3.1g
Protein: 24g
Sodium: 135mg

Chicken & Spinach Stew

Serves: 8 individuals
Preparation Time: 15 minutes
Cooking Time: 30 minutes

Ingredients:
- 2 tablespoons olive oil
- 1 medium onion, chopped
- 1 tablespoon garlic, minced
- 1 tablespoon fresh ginger, minced
- 1 teaspoon ground turmeric
- 1 teaspoon ground cumin
- 1 teaspoon ground coriander
- 1 teaspoon paprika
- 1 teaspoon cayenne powder
- 6 (4-ounce) boneless, skinless chicken thighs, trimmed and cut into 1-inch pieces
- 4 tomatoes, chopped
- 1 (14-ounce) can unsweetened coconut milk
- Salt and ground black pepper, as needed
- 3 cups fresh spinach, chopped

Directions:
1. Heat oil in a large-sized heavy-bottomed pan over medium heat and sauté the onion for approximately 3-4 minutes.
2. Add the ginger, garlic and spices and sauté for approximately 1 minute.
3. Add the chicken and cook for approximately 4-5 minutes.
4. Add the tomatoes, coconut milk, salt, and black pepper, and bring to gentle simmer.
5. Now, adjust the heat to low and simmer, covered for approximately 10–15 minutes.
6. Stir in the spinach and cook for approximately 4-5 minutes.
7. Serve hot.

Nutritional Information per Serving:
Calories: 231
Fat: 13.1g
Net Carbohydrates: 4.7g
Carbohydrates: 6.3g
Fiber: 1.6g
Sugar: 3.6g
Protein: 20.9g
Sodium: 99mg

Turkey & Squash Stew

Serves: 8 individuals
Preparation Time: 15 minutes
Cooking Time: 45 minutes

Ingredients:
- 2 tablespoons coconut oil
- 2 pounds turkey breast, cubed into 1½-inch size
- 1 onion, chopped
- 1 (2-inch) piece fresh ginger, minced
- 5 garlic cloves, minced
- 1 butternut squash, peeled and cubed
- ¼ teaspoon ground cinnamon
- ¼ teaspoon ground cumin
- 3 cups chicken bones broth
- 2 pears, cored and chopped
- Salt and ground black pepper, as needed
- 1 tablespoon fresh thyme, chopped

Directions:
1. In a large-sized heavy-bottomed pan, melt 1 tablespoon of coconut oil over medium-high heat and sear turkey cubes for approximately 3-4 minutes or until browned completely.
2. With a slotted spoon, transfer the turkey cubes into a bowl.
3. In the same pan, add the onion over medium heat and sauté for approximately 5 minutes.
4. Add ginger and garlic and sauté for approximately 1 minute.
5. Add cooked turkey, squash, cinnamon, cumin and broth and cook until boiling.
6. Now, adjust the heat to low and cook, covered for approximately 10 minutes.
7. Stir in the pears, salt and black pepper and cook, covered for approximately 20 minutes.
8. Serve hot with the topping of thyme.

Nutritional Information per Serving:
Calories: 247
Fat: 4.7g
Net Carbohydrates: 19.8g
Carbohydrates: 24.3g
Fiber: 4.5g
Sugar: 8.5g
Protein: 31.6g
Sodium: 367mg

Chicken & Beans Chili

Serves: 8 individuals
Preparation Time: 15 minutes
Cooking Time: 40 minutes

Ingredients:
- 2 tablespoons olive oil
- 1 pound boneless, skinless chicken breasts, chopped
- 1 medium onion, chopped
- 2 garlic cloves, minced
- 1 (1-inch) piece fresh ginger, minced
- 1 (4-ounce) can chopped green chiles
- 2 teaspoons dried oregano
- 2 teaspoons ground cumin
- 1½ teaspoons cayenne powder

- 28 ounces chicken bones broth
- 3 (14-ounce) cans Great Northern beans, drained, divided
- Salt and ground black pepper, as needed

Directions:
1. In a Dutch oven, heat the oil over medium heat and cook the chicken pieces and onion for approximately 3-5 minutes or until browned.
2. Add the garlic, ginger and green chiles and cook for approximately 1 minute.
3. Stir in the chiles, oregano, cumin, cayenne powder and broth and cook until boiling.
4. Meanwhile, with a potato masher, mash one can of beans until smooth.
5. Now, adjust the heat to low and stir in the pureed beans and remaining cans of beans and simmer for approximately 20-30 minutes.
6. Stir in the salt and black pepper and remove from the heat.
7. Serve hot

Nutritional Information per Serving:
Calories: 345
Fat: 9.2g
Net Carbohydrates: 23.9g
Carbohydrates: 34.9g
Fiber: 11g
Sugar: 1.4g
Protein: 31.2g
Sodium: 445mg

Turkey & Lentil Chili
Serves: 4 individuals
Preparation Time: 15 minutes
Cooking Time: 1 hour 5 minutes

Ingredients:
- 1 tablespoon olive oil
- 1 small onion, chopped
- 1 pound lean ground turkey
- 1 carrot, peeled and chopped
- 2 garlic cloves, chopped finely
- 1 tablespoon fresh ginger, minced
- 1 jalapeño pepper, seeded and chopped
- 1 (15-ounce) can diced tomatoes
- 1 cup dried red lentils
- 1 teaspoon dried oregano, crushed
- 1½ tablespoons paprika
- 2 teaspoons ground cumin
- Salt and ground black pepper, as needed
- 5 cups chicken bones broth

Directions:
1. In a large-sized Dutch oven, heat the oil over medium heat and sauté the onion for approximately 3-5 minutes.
2. Add the ground turkey and cook for approximately 4-5 minutes, breaking the lumps with a wooden spoon.

3. Add the carrot, garlic, ginger and jalapeño pepper and cook for approximately 2 minutes, stirring occasionally.
4. Stir in the remaining ingredients and cook until boiling.
5. Now, adjust the heat to low and simmer, covered for approximately 40-50 minutes, stirring occasionally.
6. Serve hot

Nutritional Information per Serving:
Calories: 378
Fat: 11.8g
Net Carbohydrates: 18.2g
Carbohydrates: 32.8g
Fiber: 14.6g
Sugar: 5.3g
Protein: 36.1g
Sodium: 934mg

Chicken & Tomato Curry
Serves: 6 individuals
Preparation Time: 15 minutes
Cooking Time: 1 hour 10 minutes

Ingredients:
- 3 tablespoons olive oil
- 1 medium onion, chopped
- 1 teaspoon ginger paste
- 1 teaspoon garlic paste
- 4-6 large fresh tomatoes, chopped finely
- 1 teaspoon ground cumin
- Pinch of ground turmeric
- 1½ teaspoons red chili powder
- 6 (4-ounce) boneless chicken breasts
- 2 cups water, divided
- 2 cardamom pods
- 2 tablespoons fresh cilantro, chopped

Directions:
1. In a large-sized saucepan, heat oil over medium heat and cook onion for approximately 8-9 minutes.
2. Add ginger and garlic and sauté for approximately 1 minute.
3. Add tomatoes and spices and stir to blend.
4. Now, adjust the heat to medium-low and cook for approximately 15-20 minutes, stirring occasionally.
5. Remove the pan of tomato mixture from heat and set aside to cool slightly.
6. In a clean blender, add tomato mixture and pulse until smooth.
7. Return the mixture to pan with chicken and ½ cup of the water over medium-high heat.
8. Cook for approximately 15-20 minutes, stirring occasionally.

9. Add cardamom pods and remaining water and now, adjust the heat to low.
10. Simmer for approximately 15-20 minutes.
11. Serve hot with the topping of cilantro.

Nutritional Information per Serving:
Calories: 310
Fat: 15.9g
Net Carbohydrates: 5.2g
Carbohydrates: 7.4g
Fiber: 2.2g
Sugar: 4g
Protein: 34.3g
Sodium: 114mg

Chicken Meatballs Curry

Serves: 4 individuals
Preparation Time: 20 minutes
Cooking Time: 30 minutes
Ingredients:
For Meatballs:
- 1 pound lean ground chicken
- 1 tablespoon onion paste
- 1 teaspoon fresh ginger paste
- 1 teaspoon garlic paste
- 1 green chili, chopped finely
- 1 tablespoon fresh cilantro leaves, chopped
- 1 teaspoon ground coriander
- ½ teaspoon cumin seeds
- ½ teaspoon red chili powder
- ½ teaspoon ground turmeric
- Salt, as needed

For Curry:
- 3 tablespoons extra-virgin olive oil
- ½ teaspoon cumin seeds
- 1 (1-inch) cinnamon stick
- 3 whole cloves
- 3 whole green cardamoms
- 1 whole black cardamom
- 2 onions, chopped
- 1 teaspoon fresh ginger, minced
- 1 teaspoon garlic, minced
- 4 whole tomatoes, chopped finely
- 2 teaspoons ground coriander
- 1 teaspoon garam masala powder
- ½ teaspoon ground nutmeg
- ½ teaspoon red chili powder
- ½ teaspoon ground turmeric
- Salt, as needed
- 1 cup water
- 2-3 tablespoons fresh cilantro, chopped

Directions:
1. For meatballs: in a large-sized bowl, add all ingredients and mix until blended thoroughly.
2. Make small equal-sized meatballs from mixture.

3. In a large-sized deep wok, heat oil over medium heat and cook the meatballs for approximately 3-5 minutes or until browned from all sides.
4. Transfer the meatballs into a bowl.
5. In the same wok, add cumin seeds, cinnamon stick, cloves, green cardamom and black cardamom and sauté for approximately 1 minute.
6. Add onions and sauté for approximately 4-5 minutes.
7. Add ginger and garlic paste and sauté for approximately 1 minute.
8. Add tomato and spices and cook, crushing with the back of spoon for approximately 2-3 minutes.
9. Add water and meatballs and cook until boiling.
10. Now, adjust the heat to low and cook for approximately 10 minutes.
11. Serve hot with the garnishing of cilantro.

Nutritional Information per Serving:
Calories: 291
Fat: 17.1g
Net Carbohydrates: 8.1g
Carbohydrates: 11.1g
Fiber: 3g
Sugar: 5.7g
Protein: 24.9g
Sodium: 179mg

Chicken in Orange Sauce

Serves: 2 individuals
Preparation Time: 15 minutes
Cooking Time: 20 minutes

Ingredients:

For Chicken:
- 1 organic egg
- ¼ cup almond flour
- ½ pound skinless, boneless chicken breasts, cut into 1-inch pieces
- 1 tablespoon coconut oil
- 1 scallion, chopped

Orange Sauce
- ¼ cup fresh orange juice
- 1 tablespoon tapioca starch
- ½ tablespoon coconut oil
- ½ teaspoon orange zest, grated finely and divided
- ½ teaspoon fresh ginger, minced
- 1 garlic clove, minced
- ¼ teaspoon red pepper flakes, crushed
- ½ tablespoon organic honey
- ½ tablespoon red boat fish sauce
- ½ teaspoon apple cider vinegar

Directions:
1. For chicken: in a shallow dish, beat the eggs.
2. In another shallow dish, place the almond flour.

3. Dip each chicken piece in eggs and then coat with almond flour evenly.
4. In a Dutch oven, melt the coconut oil over medium heat and cook the chicken pieces for 5 minutes or until golden brown from all sides.
5. With a slotted spoon, transfer the cooked chicken pieces onto a plate.
6. For sauce: in a small-sized bowl, blend together orange juice and tapioca starch.
7. In the same pan, melt the coconut oil over medium heat and sauté half of orange zest, ginger, garlic and red pepper flakes for approximately 1 minute.
8. Stir in honey, fish sauce and vinegar and cook for approximately 1 minute.
9. Add orange juice mixture and cook until boiling, stirring continuously.
10. Now, adjust the heat to low and simmer for approximately 1-2 minutes, stirring continuously.
11. Add in the cooked chicken pieces and cook for approximately 4-5 minutes.
12. Serve hot with the garnishing of scallion and remaining orange zest.

Nutritional Information per Serving:
Calories: 397
Fat: 23.6g
Net Carbohydrates: 14.7g
Carbohydrates: 16.7g
Fiber: 2g
Sugar: 8.1g
Protein: 31.9g
Sodium: 421mg

Chicken with Pineapple

Serves: 4 individuals
Preparation Time: 15 minutes
Cooking Time: 13 minutes

Ingredients:
- 2 tablespoons coconut oil
- 1½ pounds boneless chicken breasts, cut into thin slices
- 1 onion, chopped
- 2 garlic cloves, minced
- 1 (1-inch) piece fresh ginger, minced
- 20 ounces pineapple, cut into chunks
- 1 large bell pepper, seeded and chopped
- ¼ cup fresh pineapple juice
- ¼ cup coconut aminos
- Salt and ground black pepper, as needed

Directions:
1. In a large-sized wok, melt coconut oil over high heat and stir fry the chicken slices for approximately 3-4 minutes.
2. Transfer the chicken slices into a bowl.
3. In the same wok, melt the remaining coconut oil over medium heat and cook onion, garlic and ginger for approximately 2 minutes.

4. Stir in pineapple and bell pepper and stir fry for approximately 3 minutes.
5. Stir in the cooked chicken slices, pineapple juice and coconut aminos and cook for approximately 3-4 minutes.
6. Serve hot.

Nutritional Information per Serving:
Calories: 490
Fat: 19.7g
Net Carbohydrates: 23.9g
Carbohydrates: 26.9g
Fiber: 3g
Sugar: 16.7g
Protein: 50.7g
Sodium: 206mg

Chicken with Broccoli & Spinach

Serves: 4 individuals
Preparation Time: 15 minutes
Cooking Time: 13 minutes

Ingredients:
- 13 ounces unsweetened coconut milk
- 1 teaspoon fresh ginger, grated
- 1½ teaspoons curry powder
- 2 tablespoons coconut oil, divided
- 1 pound boneless chicken breasts, sliced thinly
- 1 large onion, chopped
- 2 cups broccoli florets
- 1 large bunch fresh spinach, chopped

Directions:
1. In a bowl, blend together coconut milk, ginger and curry powder. Set aside.
2. In a large-sized wok, melt 1 tablespoon of coconut oil over medium-high heat.
3. Add chicken and stir fry for approximately 3-4 minutes or until golden brown.
4. Transfer chicken into a bowl.
5. In the same wok, heat the remaining oil over medium-high heat and the onion for approximately 2 minutes.
6. Add broccoli and stir fry for approximately 3 minutes.
7. Add chicken, spinach and coconut mixture and stir fry for approximately 3-4 minutes.
8. Serve hot.

Nutritional Information per Serving:
Calories: 473
Fat: 28.6g
Net Carbohydrates: 8.9g
Carbohydrates: 13.7g
Fiber: 4.8g
Sugar: 5.2g
Protein: 39g
Sodium: 233mg

Chicken Casserole

Serves: 10 individuals
Preparation Time: 20 minutes
Cooking Time: 1 hour 20 minutes

Ingredients:
- 2 tablespoons coconut oil, divided
- 3 pounds bone-in chicken thighs and drumsticks
- Salt and ground black pepper, as needed
- 3 carrots, peeled and sliced
- 1 onion, chopped finely
- 2 garlic cloves, chopped finely
- 2 tablespoons fresh ginger root, chopped finely
- 2 teaspoons ground cumin
- 1 teaspoon ground coriander
- 12 teaspoon ground cinnamon
- ½ teaspoon ground turmeric
- 1 teaspoon paprika
- ¼ teaspoon cayenne powder
- 1 (28-ounce) can diced tomatoes with liquid
- 1 red bell pepper, seeded and cut into thin strips
- ½ cup fresh parsley leaves, minced
- Salt, as needed
- 1 head cauliflower, grated to a rice-like consistency
- 1 lemon, sliced thinly

Directions:
1. Preheat your oven to 375 °F.
2. In a large-sized saucepan, melt 1 tablespoon of coconut oil over high heat and cook chicken pieces for approximately 3-5 minutes per side or until golden brown.
3. Transfer the chicken pieces into a bowl.
4. In the same pan, sauté the carrot, onion, garlic and ginger for approximately 4-5 minutes over medium heat.
5. Add in the spices and remaining coconut oil and stir to blend.
6. Add chicken, tomatoes, bell pepper, parsley and salt and simmer for approximately 3-5 minutes.
7. In the bottom of a 13x9-inch rectangular baking dish, spread the cauliflower rice evenly.
8. Place chicken mixture over cauliflower rice evenly and top with lemon slices.
9. With a piece of foil, cover the baking dish and bake for approximately 35 minutes.
10. Uncover the baking dish and bake for approximately 25 minutes.
11. Remove the baking dish from oven and set aside for approximately 5 minutes before serving.

Nutritional Information per Serving
Calories: 265
Fat: 16.8g
Net Carbohydrates: 7.2g
Carbohydrates: 11.4g

Fiber: 4.2g
Sugar: 4.9g
Protein: 20g
Sodium: 341mg

Turkey with Bell Pepper & Asparagus

Serves: 4 individuals
Preparation Time: 15 minutes
Cooking Time: 15 minutes

Ingredients:
- 4 garlic cloves, minced
- 3 tablespoons coconut aminos
- 1/8 teaspoon red pepper flakes, crushed
- 1/8 teaspoon ground ginger
- Ground black pepper, as needed
- 1 bunch asparagus, trimmed and halved
- 2 tablespoons olive oil, divided
- 1 pound boneless turkey breast, sliced thinly
- 1 red bell pepper, seeded and sliced
- 3 tablespoons water
- 2 teaspoons arrowroot powder

Directions:
1. In a bowl, blend together garlic, coconut aminos, red pepper flakes, crushed, ground ginger and black pepper. Set aside.
2. In a pan of boiling water, cook the asparagus for approximately 2 minutes.
3. Drain the asparagus and rinse under cold water.
4. In a large-sized wok, heat 1 tablespoon of oil over medium-high heat and stir fry the turkey slices for approximately 3-5 minutes.
5. With a slotted spoon, transfer the turkey slices into a bowl.
6. In the same wok, heat the remaining oil over medium heat and stir fry the asparagus and bell pepper for approximately 3-4 minutes.
7. Meanwhile, in a bowl, blend together water and arrowroot powder.
8. In the wok, add the cooked turkey slices, garlic mixture and arrowroot mixture and cook for approximately 3-4 minutes or until desired thickness, stirring frequently.
9. Serve hot.

Nutritional Information per Serving:
Calories: 239
Fat: 7.7g
Net Carbohydrates: 7.9g
Carbohydrates: 10.2g
Fiber: 2.3g
Sugar: 3.1g
Protein: 30.4g
Sodium: 71mg

Ground Turkey with Greens

Serves: 4 individuals
Preparation Time: 10 minutes
Cooking Time: 15 minutes

Ingredients:
- 1 tablespoon olive oil
- ½ of white onion, chopped
- 2 garlic cloves, chopped finely
- 1 jalapeño pepper, chopped finely
- 1 pound lean ground turkey
- 1 teaspoon ground coriander
- 1 teaspoon ground cumin
- ½ teaspoon ground turmeric
- ½ teaspoon ground ginger
- ½ teaspoon ground cinnamon
- ½ teaspoon ground fennel seeds
- Salt and ground black pepper, as needed
- 8 fresh cherry tomatoes, quartered
- 1½ pounds collard greens, stemmed and chopped
- 1 teaspoon fresh lemon juice

Directions:
1. In a large-sized wok, heat oil over medium heat and cook onion for approximately 4 minutes.
2. Add garlic and jalapeño pepper and sauté for approximately 1 minute.
3. Add turkey and spices and cook for approximately 6 minutes breaking into pieces with the spoon.
4. Stir in tomatoes and greens and cook, stirring gently for approximately 4 minutes.
5. Stir in lemon juice and remove from heat.
6. Serve hot.

Nutritional Information per Serving:
Calories: 256
Fat: 13.1g
Net Carbohydrates: 6.5g
Carbohydrates: 13.1g
Fiber: 6.6g
Sugar: 1.4g
Protein: 26.7g
Sodium: 156mg

Ground Turkey with Green Peas

Serves: 2 individuals
Preparation Time: 15 minutes
Cooking Time: 40 minutes

Ingredients:
- 1 tablespoon coconut oil
- 1 dried red chili
- 1 cinnamon stick
- 1 green cardamom pod
- ¼ teaspoon cumin seeds
- 1 small red onion, chopped
- 1 (¼-inch) piece fresh ginger, minced
- 2 garlic cloves, minced
- ½ teaspoon ground coriander
- ¼ teaspoon garam masala powder
- ¼ teaspoon ground cumin
- ½ teaspoon ground turmeric
- 1 bay leaf
- ½ pound lean ground turkey
- 1/3 cup tomatoes, chopped
- 1 cup water
- ½ cup fresh green peas, shelled
- 2 tablespoons fat-free plain Greek yogurt, whipped
- 2 tablespoons fresh cilantro, chopped
- Salt and ground black pepper, as needed

Directions:
1. In a Dutch oven, melt coconut oil over medium-high heat and sauté the red chilies, cinnamon stick, cardamom pods and cumin seeds for approximately 30 seconds.
2. Add the onion and sauté for approximately 3-4 minutes.
3. Add the ginger, garlic cloves and spices and sauté for approximately 30 seconds.
4. Add the beef and cook for approximately 5 minutes.
5. Add the tomatoes and cook for approximately 10 minutes.
6. Stir in the water and green peas and cook, covered for approximately 25-30 minutes.
7. Stir in the yogurt, cilantro, salt and black pepper and cook for approximately 4-5 minutes
8. Discard the bay leaves and serve hot.

Nutritional Information per Serving:
Calories: 196
Net Carbohydrates: 5.8g
Fat: 9.6g
Carbohydrates: 8.2g
Fiber: 2.4g
Sugar: 3.1g
Protein: 20g
Sodium: 104mg

Ground Turkey with Cabbage

Serves: 4 individuals
Preparation Time: 15 minutes
Cooking Time: 12 minutes

Ingredients:
- 1 tablespoon olive oil
- 1 onion, sliced thinly
- 2 teaspoons fresh ginger, minced
- 4 garlic cloves, minced
- 1 pound lean ground turkey
- 1½ tablespoons red boat fish sauce
- 2 tablespoons fresh lime juice
- 1 small head purple cabbage, shredded
- 2 tablespoons peanut butter
- ½ cup fresh cilantro, chopped

Directions:
1. In a large-sized wok, heat oil over medium heat and cook onion, ginger and garlic for approximately 4 5 minutes.
2. Add turkey and cook for approximately 7-8 minutes, breaking into pieces with the spoon.
3. Drain off the excess liquid from the wok.
4. Stir in fish sauce and lime juice and cook for approximately 1 minute.
5. Add cabbage and cook for approximately 4-5 minutes or until desired doneness.
6. Stir in peanut butter and cilantro and cook for approximately 1 minute.
7. Serve hot.

Nutritional Information per Serving:
Calories: 309
Fat: 15.9g
Net Carbohydrates: 10.5g
Carbohydrates: 16.3g
Fiber: 5.8g
Sugar: 7.7g
Protein: 28.7g
Sodium: 717mg

Duck with Bok Choy

Serves: 6 individuals
Preparation Time: 15 minutes
Cooking Time: 12 minutes

Ingredients:
- 2 tablespoons coconut oil
- 1 onion, sliced thinly
- 2 teaspoons fresh ginger, grated finely
- 2 garlic cloves, minced
- 1 tablespoon fresh orange zest, grated finely
- ¼ cup chicken broth
- 2/3 cup fresh orange juice
- 1 pound cooked duck meat, chopped
- 1 pound bok choy leaves
- 1 orange, peeled, seeded and segmented

Directions:
1. In a large-sized wok, melt coconut oil over medium heat and cook onion, ginger and garlic for approximately 3 minutes.
2. Add ginger and garlic and sauté for approximately 1-2 minutes.
3. Add in orange zest, broth and orange juice and stir to blend.
4. Add duck meat and cook for approximately 1-2 minutes.
5. Add in the bok choy and cook for approximately 3-4 minutes.
6. Serve with the garnishing of orange segments.

Nutritional Information per Serving:
Calories: 246
Fat: 13.5g
Net Carbohydrates: 9.2g
Carbohydrates: 11.7g
Fiber: 2.5g
Sugar: 7.4g
Protein: 20.5g
Sodium: 156mg

CHAPTER 6:
Fish & Seafood Recipes

Spicy Salmon Soup

Serves: 6 individuals
Preparation Time: 15 minutes
Cooking Time: 35 minutes

Ingredients:

- 2 pounds salmon fillet, cut into chunks
- 1½ teaspoon ground coriander
- 1 teaspoon ground cumin
- ½ teaspoon ground turmeric
- ½ teaspoon red pepper flakes
- ½ teaspoon paprika
- Salt and ground black pepper, as needed
- 3 tablespoons olive oil
- 2 celery stalks, chopped
- 1 medium red onion, chopped
- 1 bell pepper, seeded and chopped
- 4 garlic cloves, minced
- 1 (28-ounce) can whole peeled tomatoes
- 5½ cups chicken bones broth
- 2 tablespoons fresh lemon juice
- ¼ cup fresh parsley, chopped

Directions:

1. In a bowl, add salmon chunks, spices, salt and black pepper and toss to combine.
2. Transfer the salmon chunks onto a plate, reserving the remaining spice mixture.
3. In a large-sized Dutch oven, heat oil over medium-high heat and sauté the celery, onions, bell peppers and garlic for approximately 3-4 minutes.
4. Add in the reserved spice mixture and sauté for approximately 1 minute.
5. Add the tomatoes and broth and cook until boiling.
6. Adjust the heat to medium-low and simmer, partially covered for approximately 20 minutes.
7. Add in the salmon chunks and cook for approximately 4-5 minutes.
8. Remove the soup pan from heat and stir in the lemon juice.
9. Serve hot with the garnishing of parsley.

Nutritional Information per Serving:

Calories: 339
Fat: 16.9g
Net Carbohydrates: 7.2g
Carbohydrates: 9.9g
Fiber: 2.7g
Sugar: 5.6g
Protein: 39.5g
Sodium: 197mg

Salmon & Cabbage Soup

Serves: 4 individuals
Preparation Time: 15 minutes
Cooking Time: 30 minutes

Ingredients:

- 2 tablespoons olive oil
- 1 shallot, chopped
- 2 small garlic cloves, minced
- 1 tablespoon fresh ginger, minced
- 1 jalapeño pepper, chopped
- 1 large cabbage head, chopped
- 4 cups homemade vegetable broth
- 3 (4-ounce) boneless salmon fillets, cubed
- ¼ cup fresh cilantro, minced
- 2 tablespoons fresh lemon juice
- Salt and ground black pepper, as needed
- 3 tablespoons fresh parsley, chopped

Directions:

1. In a large-sized soup pan, heat oil over medium heat and sauté shallot and garlic for 2-3 minutes.
2. Add cabbage and sauté for approximately 3-4 minutes.
3. Add broth and cook until boiling over high heat.
4. Now, adjust the heat to medium-low and simmer for approximately 10 minutes.
5. Add salmon and cook for approximately 5-6 minutes.
6. Stir in the cilantro, lemon juice, salt and black pepper and cook for approximately 1-2 minutes.
7. Serve hot with the topping of dill.

Nutritional Information per Serving:

Calories: 260
Fat: 12.7g
Net Carbohydrates: 15.5g
Carbohydrates: 21g
Fiber: 5.5g
Sugar: 13.4g
Protein: 19.9g
Sodium: 94mg

Cod Soup

Serves: 4 individuals
Preparation Time: 15 minutes
Cooking Time: 37 minutes

Ingredients:
- 1 teaspoon olive oil
- ¼ cup fresh parsley, chopped
- 2 garlic cloves, minced
- 1 teaspoon fresh ginger, minced
- 3 tomatoes, chopped
- 10 canned oil-packed anchovies, minced
- Salt and ground black pepper, as needed
- 6 cups homemade vegetable broth
- 1 pound cod fillets, chopped
- 3-4 scallions, chopped

Directions:
1. In a large-sized soup pan, heat olive oil over medium heat and sauté the parsley, garlic and ginger for approximately 1 minute.
2. Add the tomatoes, anchovies, salt, black pepper and broth and stir to blend.
3. Now, adjust the heat to high and cook until boiling.
4. Now, adjust the heat to medium-low and simmer, covered for approximately 15-20 minutes.
5. Add in the halibut and scallions and cook, covered for approximately 8-10 minutes.
6. Serve hot.

Nutritional Information per Serving:
Calories: 199
Fat: 3.5g
Net Carbohydrates: 7g
Carbohydrates: 10.2g
Fiber: 3.2g
Sugar: 5.8g
Protein: 30.1g
Sodium: 909mg

Shrimp & Mushroom Soup

Serves: 6 individuals
Preparation Time: 15 minutes
Cooking Time: 30 minutes

Ingredients:
- 1 tablespoon olive oil
- 1 small onion, chopped
- 1 tablespoon lemongrass, minced
- 1 tablespoon fresh ginger, minced
- 2 garlic cloves, minced
- 1 tablespoon red curry paste
- 3 cups chicken bones broth
- 1 tablespoon red boat fish sauce
- 2 (14-ounce) cans full-fat coconut milk
- 8 ounces fresh shiitake mushrooms, sliced
- 1 pound medium shrimp, peeled and deveined
- 1½ tablespoons fresh lime juice
- 2 teaspoons lime zest, grated
- Salt, as needed

Directions:
1. In a large-sized soup pan, heat the oil over medium heat and sauté the onion for approximately 5-7 minutes.
2. Stir in the lemongrass, ginger, garlic and curry paste and sauté for approximately 1 minute.
3. Stir in the broth and fish sauce and simmer for approximately 10 minutes.
4. Add the coconut milk and stir to blend.
5. Add in the mushrooms and cook for approximately 5 minutes.
6. Add the shrimp and cook for approximately 5 minutes.
7. Stir in the lime juice, zest and juice and salt and serve hot.

Nutritional Information per Serving:
Calories: 404
Fat: 29.7g
Net Carbohydrates: 9g
Carbohydrates: 9.8g
Fiber: 0.8g
Sugar: 3.6g
Protein: 23.8g
Sodium: 990mg

Poached Salmon

Serves: 3 individuals
Preparation Time: 10 minutes
Cooking Time: 17 minutes

Ingredients:
- 3 garlic cloves, crushed
- 1½ teaspoons fresh ginger, grated finely
- 1/3 cup fresh orange juice
- 3 tablespoons coconut aminos
- 3 (6-ounce) salmon fillets

Directions:
1. In a medium-sized bowl, add garlic, ginger, orange juice and coconut aminos and stir to blend.
2. In the bottom of a large-sized saucepan, place the salmon fillets and top with ginger mixture evenly.
3. Set aside for approximately 15 minutes.
4. Place the pan over high heat and cook until boiling.
5. Now, adjust the heat to low and simmer, covered for approximately 10-12 minutes or until desired doneness.
6. Serve hot.

Nutritional Information per Serving:
Calories: 260
Fat: 10.6g
Net Carbohydrates: 7.3g
Carbohydrates: 7.5g
Fiber: 0.2g
Sugar: 2.4g
Protein: 33.5g
Sodium: 93mg

Spiced Salmon

Serves: 6 individuals
Preparation Time: 10 minutes
Cooking Time: 8 minutes

Ingredients:
- ½ tablespoon ground ginger
- ½ tablespoon ground coriander
- ½ tablespoon ground cumin
- ½ teaspoon paprika
- ¼ teaspoon cayenne powder
- Salt, as needed
- 1 tablespoon fresh orange juice
- 1 tablespoon coconut oil, melted
- 1½-2 pounds salmon fillets
- Olive oil cooking spray

Directions:
1. In a large-sized bowl, add all ingredients except salmon and mix until a paste forms.
2. Add salmon and coat with mixture generously.
3. Refrigerate to marinate for approximately 30 minutes.
4. Preheat the gas grill to high heat with the lid closed for at least 10 minutes.
5. Grease the grill grate with cooking spray and place the salmon fillets, skin-side down.
6. Cover the grill with the lid and cook for approximately 3-4 minutes per side.
7. Serve hot.

Nutritional Information per Serving:
Calories: 175
Fat: 9.5g
Net Carbohydrates: 0.8g
Carbohydrates: 1g
Fiber: 0.2g
Sugar: 0.3g
Protein: 22.2g
Sodium: 78mg

Sweet & Sour Salmon

Serves: 4 individuals
Preparation Time: 10 minutes
Cooking Time: 12 minutes

Ingredients:

- 2 garlic cloves, crushed
- 2 tablespoons fresh ginger, grated finely
- 2 tablespoons organic honey
- 2 tablespoons coconut aminos
- 2 tablespoons fresh lime juice
- 3 tablespoons olive oil
- 2 tablespoons black sesame seeds
- 1 tablespoon white sesame seeds
- 1 pound boneless salmon fillets
- 1/3 cup scallion, chopped

Directions:

1. In a baking dish, blend together all ingredients except for the salmon and scallion.
2. Add salmon and coat with mixture generously.
3. Refrigerate to marinate for approximately 40-45 minutes.
4. Preheat the broiler of oven.
5. Place the baking dish in the oven and broil for approximately 10-12 minutes.
6. Remove the baking dish from oven and transfer the salmon fillets onto a serving platter.
7. Top the salmon fillets with the pan sauce and garnish with scallion.
8. Serve immediately.

Nutritional Information per Serving:

Calories: 324
Fat: 20.9g
Net Carbohydrates:11.8
Carbohydrates: 12.9g
Fiber: 1.1g
Sugar: 8.9g
Protein: 23.5g
Sodium: 61mg

Cheesy Salmon Parcel

Serves: 4 individuals
Preparation Time: 10 minutes
Cooking Time: 25 minutes

Ingredients:

- 2 garlic cloves, crushed
- 1 teaspoon dried dill weed, crushed
- Salt and ground black pepper, as needed
- 4 (5-ounce) salmon fillets
- ½ cup low-fat cheddar cheese, shredded
- 4 scallions, chopped

Directions:

1. Preheat your oven to 450 °F.
2. In a bowl, blend together garlic, dill weed, salt and black pepper.
3. Rub the salmon fillets with garlic mixture evenly.
4. Arrange the salmon fillets over a large-sized piece of foil and then fold it to seal.
5. Place the salmon parcel onto a baking sheet and bake for approximately 20 minutes.
6. Now, unfold the parcel and top the salmon fillets with cheese and scallions.
7. Bake for approximately 5 minutes.
8. Serve hot.

Nutritional Information per Serving:

Calories: 252
Fat: 13.5g
Net Carbohydrates: 1.4g
Carbohydrates: 1.9g
Fiber: 0.5g
Sugar: 0.4g
Protein: 31.4g
Sodium: 192mg

Salmon in Spicy Yogurt Sauce

Serves: 5 individuals
Preparation Time: 15 minutes
Cooking Time: 35 minutes

Ingredients:

- 5 (4-ounce) salmon fillets
- 1½ teaspoons ground turmeric, divided
- Salt, as needed
- 3 tablespoons coconut oil, divided
- 1 (1-inch) stick cinnamon, pounded roughly
- 3-4 green cardamom, pounded roughly
- 4-5 whole cloves, pounded roughly
- 2 bay leaves
- 1 onion, chopped finely
- 1 teaspoon garlic paste
- 1½ teaspoons fresh ginger paste
- 3-4 green chilies, halved
- 1 teaspoon red chili powder
- ¾ cup fat-free plain Greek yogurt
- ¾ cup water
- ¼ cup fresh cilantro, chopped

Directions:

1. In a bowl, season the salmon with ½ teaspoon of the turmeric and salt and set aside.
2. In a large-sized, non-stick wok, melt 1 tablespoon of coconut oil over medium heat and cook salmon fillets for approximately 2-3 minutes per side.
3. Transfer the salmon fillets into a bowl.
4. In the same wok, melt remaining oil over medium heat and sauté cinnamon, green cardamom, whole cloves and bay leaves for approximately 1 minute.
5. Add onion and sauté for approximately 4-5 minutes.
6. Add garlic paste, ginger paste, green chilies and sauté for approximately 2 minutes.
7. Now, adjust the heat to medium-low.
8. Add remaining turmeric, red chili powder and salt and sauté for approximately 1 minute.
9. Meanwhile, in a bowl, add yogurt and water and whisk until smooth.
10. Now, adjust the heat to low and slowly, add the yogurt mixture, stirring continuously.
11. Cover the wok and cook for approximately 15 minutes.
12. Add in the salmon fillets and simmer for approximately 5 minutes.
13. Serve hot with the topping of cilantro.

Nutritional Information per Serving
Calories: 313
Fat: 18.3g
Net Carbohydrates: 1.3g
Carbohydrates: 1.4g
Fiber: 0.1g
Sugar: 1g
Protein: 34g
Sodium: 149mg

Salmon with Peach

Serves: 4 individuals
Preparation Time: 15 minutes
Cooking Time: 12 minutes

Ingredients:

- Olive oil cooking spray
- 4 (5-ounce) salmon fillets
- Salt and ground black pepper, as needed
- 3 peaches, pitted and cut into wedges
- 2 medium red onions, cut into wedges
- 1 tablespoon fresh ginger, minced
- 1 teaspoon fresh thyme leaves, minced
- 3 tablespoons olive oil
- 1 tablespoon balsamic vinegar

Directions:

1. Preheat the grill to medium heat.
2. Grease the grill grate with cooking spray.
3. Rub the salmon fillets with salt and black pepper evenly.
4. In a bowl, add peaches, onion, salt and black pepper and toss to combine.
5. Place the salmon fillets onto the grill and cook for approximately 5-6 minutes per side.
6. Place peaches and onions onto the grill with salmon fillets and cook for approximately 3-4 minutes per side.
7. Meanwhile, in a bowl, add remaining ingredients and mix until a smooth paste forms.
8. Place ginger mixture over salmon filets evenly and serve with peaches and onions.

Nutritional Information per Serving:
Calories: 350
Fat: 19.7g
Net Carbohydrates: 13.6g
Carbohydrates: 16.8g
Fiber: 3.2g
Sugar: 12.9g
Protein: 29.3g
Sodium: 165mg

Tilapia Parcel

Serves: 3 individuals
Preparation Time: 10 minutes
Cooking Time: 10 minutes

Ingredients:

- 2 tablespoons garlic, minced
- 1 tablespoon fresh turmeric, grated finely
- 1 tablespoon fresh ginger root, grated finely
- 2 tablespoons fresh lime juice
- 2 tablespoons coconut aminos
- 2 tablespoons olive oil
- 1 bunch fresh cilantro, chopped
- 3 (6-ounce) tilapia fillets

Directions:

1. In a clean food processor, add garlic, turmeric, ginger, lime juice, coconut aminos and olive oil and pulse until smooth.
2. Transfer the ginger mixture into a bowl with cilantro and mix well.
3. Add tilapia fillets and coat with the mixture generously.
4. Place each tilapia fillet in the center of a piece of foil.
5. Wrap the foil around fish to form a parcel.
6. Arrange a steamer basket in a saucepan of boiling water.
7. Place the parcels in steamer basket and steam, covered for approximately 10 minutes.
8. Serve hot.

Nutritional Information per Serving:

Calories: 241
Fat: 10.9g
Net Carbohydrates: 4.2g
Carbohydrates: 4.4g
Fiber: 0.2g
Sugar: 0.1g
Protein: 32.1g
Sodium: 73mg

Tilapia with Veggies

Serves: 2 individuals
Preparation Time: 15 minutes
Cooking Time: 15 minutes

Ingredients:

- 1 (8-ounce) tilapia fillet, cubed
- ¼ teaspoon ginger paste
- ¼ teaspoon garlic paste
- 1 teaspoon red chili powder
- Salt, as needed
- 1 tablespoon coconut vinegar
- 1 tablespoon extra-virgin olive oil, divided
- ½ cup fresh mushrooms, sliced
- 1 small onion, quartered
- ½ cup bell pepper, seeded and cubed
- 2-3 scallions, chopped
- 1 teaspoon red boat fish sauce

Directions:

1. In a bowl, blend together tilapia, ginger, garlic, chili powder and salt and set aside for approximately 20 minutes.
2. In a non-stick wok, heat 1 teaspoon of oil over medium-high heat and sear the tilapia cubes for approximately 3-4 minutes or until golden from all sides.
3. In another wok, heat remaining oil over medium heat and stir fry the mushrooms and onion for approximately 5-7 minutes.
4. Add bell pepper and tilapia cubes and stir fry for approximately 2 minutes.
5. Add scallion and fish sauce and stir fry for bout 1-2 minutes.
6. Serve hot.

Nutritional Information per Serving:

Calories: 193
Fat: 8.5g
Net Carbohydrates: 6g
Carbohydrates: 8.2g
Fiber: 2.2g
Sugar: 3.7g
Protein: 23.5g
Sodium: 385mg

Crispy Cod

Serves: 4 individuals
Preparation Time: 15 minutes
Cooking Time: 15 minutes

Ingredients:

- 1 large bell pepper, seeded and sliced
- 2 large organic eggs
- 1/3 cup blanched almond flour
- ¼ teaspoon dried dill weed, crushed
- ½ teaspoon garlic powder
- 1/8 teaspoon ground turmeric
- Ground black pepper, as needed
- 4 (5-ounce) cod fillets

Directions:

1. Preheat your oven to 350 °F.
2. Line a large-sized rimmed baking dish with parchment paper.
3. Arrange the bell pepper slices into prepared baking dish.
4. In a shallow dish, whisk the eggs.
5. In another shallow dish, blend together almond flour, dill weed, garlic powder, turmeric and black pepper.
6. Coat the cod fillets in egg and then roll into flour mixture evenly.
7. Place the cod fillets over bell pepper slices.
8. Bake for approximately 15 minutes.

9. Serve hot.

Nutritional Information per Serving:
Calories: 214
Fat: 8.5g
Net Carbohydrates: 3.3g
Carbohydrates: 4.8g
Fiber: 1.5g
Sugar: 2.1g
Protein: 30.8g
Sodium: 125mg

Spicy Cod
Serves: 4 individuals
Preparation Time: 10 minutes
Cooking Time: 14 minutes

Ingredients:
- Olive oil cooking spray
- ¼ cup fat-free plain Greek yogurt
- ½ teaspoon ground coriander
- ½ teaspoon ground turmeric
- ½ teaspoon ground ginger
- ¼ teaspoon cayenne powder
- Salt and ground black pepper, as needed
- 4 (6-ounce) skinless cod fillets

Directions:
1. Preheat the broiler of your oven.
2. Grease a broiler pan with cooking spray.
3. In a large-sized bowl, blend together yogurt, spices, salt and black pepper.
4. Arrange salmon fillets onto the prepared broiler pan in a single layer.
5. Place the yogurt mixture over each fillet evenly.
6. Broil for approximately 12-14 minutes.
7. Serve immediately.

Nutritional Information per Serving:
Calories: 146
Fat: 1.6g
Net Carbohydrates: 1.4g
Carbohydrates: 1.5g
Fiber: 0.1g
Sugar: 0g
Protein: 31g
Sodium: 156mg

Shrimp with Broccoli

Serves: 6 individuals
Preparation Time: 15 minutes
Cooking Time: 12 minutes

Ingredients:
- 2 tablespoons coconut oil, divided
- 4 cups broccoli, chopped
- 2 pounds large shrimp, peeled and deveined
- 2 garlic cloves, minced
- 1 (1-inch) piece fresh ginger, minced
- Salt and ground black pepper, as needed

Directions:
1. In a large-sized wok, melt 1 tablespoon of coconut oil over medium-high heat and cook the broccoli for approximately 3-4 minutes.
2. With the spoon, push the broccoli to the sides of pan.
3. In the center of wok, add remaining coconut oil and let it melt.
4. Add shrimp and cook for approximately 2-3 minutes, tossing occasionally.
5. Add in garlic, ginger, salt and black pepper and cook for approximately 2-3 minutes, stirring occasionally.
6. Serve hot.

Nutritional Information per Serving:
Calories: 241
Fat: 7.3g
Net Carbohydrates: 5.1g
Carbohydrates: 6.7g
Fiber: 1.6g
Sugar: 1g
Protein: 36.2g
Sodium: 416mg

Shrimp & Tomato Curry

Serves: 4 individuals
Preparation Time: 15 minutes
Cooking Time: 16 minutes

Ingredients:
- 2 tablespoons peanut oil
- ½ sweet onion, minced
- 2 garlic cloves, minced
- 1½ teaspoons ground turmeric
- 1 teaspoon ground cumin
- 1 teaspoon ground ginger
- 1 teaspoon paprika
- ½ teaspoon red chili powder
- 1 (14-ounce) can unsweetened coconut milk
- 1 (14 ½-ounce) can diced tomatoes
- Salt, as needed
- 1 pound cooked shrimp, peeled and deveined

- 2 tablespoons fresh cilantro, chopped

Directions:
1. In a large-sized wok, heat oil over medium-low heat and cook onion for approximately 5 minutes.
2. Add garlic and spices and sauté for approximately 1 minute.
3. Add coconut milk, tomatoes and salt and simmer for approximately 4-5 minutes, stirring occasionally.
4. Stir in the shrimp and cilantro and simmer for approximately 4-5 minutes.
5. Serve hot.

Nutritional Information per Serving:
Calories: 386
Fat: 23.1g
Net Carbohydrates: 00g
Carbohydrates: 13g
Fiber: 2.6g
Sugar: 6g
Protein: 28.7g
Sodium: 358mg

Shrimp, Fruit & Bell Pepper Curry

Serves: 6 individuals
Preparation Time: 15 minutes
Cooking Time: 15 minutes

Ingredients:
- 2 tablespoons coconut oil
- ½ cup onion, sliced thinly
- 1½ pound shrimp, peeled and deveined
- ½ of red bell pepper, seeded and sliced thinly
- 1 mango, peeled, pitted and sliced
- 8 ounce can of pineapple tidbits with unsweetened juice
- 1 cup unsweetened coconut milk
- 1 tablespoon red curry paste
- 2 tablespoons fish sauce
- 2 tablespoons fresh cilantro, chopped

Directions:
1. In a large-sized, non-stick saucepan, melt coconut oil over medium-high heat and cook onion for approximately 3-4 minutes.
2. Add in shrimp and cook for approximately 2 minutes per side.
3. Add bell peppers and cook for approximately 3-4 minutes.
4. Add remaining ingredients except for cilantro and simmer for approximately 5 minutes.
5. Serve hot with the topping of cilantro.

Nutritional Information per Serving
Calories: 311
Fat: 14g
Net Carbohydrates: 17g
Carbohydrates: 19.7g
Fiber: 2.7g
Sugar: 13.8g
Protein: 27.9g
Sodium: 310mg

Prawns & Veggies Curry

Serves: 5 individuals
Preparation Time: 15 minutes
Cooking Time: 11 minutes

Ingredients:
- 2 teaspoons coconut oil
- 1½ medium onions, sliced
- 1 tablespoon fresh ginger, grated finely
- 2 medium green bell peppers, sliced
- 3 medium carrots, peeled and sliced
- 1½ pound prawns, peeled and deveined
- 3 garlic cloves, minced
- 2½ teaspoons curry powder
- 1½ tablespoons fish sauce
- 1 cup unsweetened coconut milk
- Water, as needed
- 2 tablespoons fresh lime juice
- Salt, as needed

Directions:
1. In a large-sized wok, melt coconut oil over medium-high heat and cook onion for approximately 2-3 minutes.
2. Add ginger, bell pepper and carrots and stir fry for approximately 2-3 minutes.
3. Add prawns, garlic, curry powder and fish sauce and stir fry for approximately 30-60 seconds.
4. Add coconut milk and a splash of water and cook for approximately 3-4 minutes.
5. Stir in lime juice and salt and serve hot.

Nutritional Information per Serving:
Calories: 305
Fat: 11.1g
Net Carbohydrates: 12.9g
Carbohydrates: 15.7g
Fiber: 2.8g
Sugar: 7.1g
Protein: 32.8g
Sodium: 824mg

Scallops with Veggies

Serves: 2 individuals
Preparation Time: 15 minutes
Cooking Time: 15 minutes

Ingredients:
- ¾ cup chicken bones broth, divided
- 1 cup carrot, peeled and chopped
- 1 cup celery chopped
- 1½ cups green beans, trimmed and chopped
- ¾ of green apple, cored and chopped
- ½ teaspoon fresh ginger root, grated finely
- 1 teaspoon ground cardamom
- Salt and ground black pepper, as needed
- 2 teaspoons olive oil
- 8 ounces sea scallops, side muscles removed

Directions:
1. In a large-sized wok, add ¼ cup of broth and cook until boiling.
2. Add in the carrots and celery and cook for approximately 4-5 minutes.
3. Stir in green beans, apple, ginger, cardamom, salt, black pepper and remaining broth and cook for approximately 3-4 minutes.
4. Meanwhile in a frying pan, heat oil and cook the scallops for approximately 2-3 minutes per side.
5. Transfer the scallops into the wok with veggie mixture and stir to blend.
6. Serve immediately.

Nutritional Information per Serving:
Calories: 326
Fat: 6.7g
Net Carbohydrates: 29g
Carbohydrates: 43.8g
Fiber: 14.8g
Sugar: 16.6g
Protein: 27.5g
Sodium: 644mg

Squid with Veggies

Serves: 4 individuals
Preparation Time: 15 minutes
Cooking Time: 10 minutes

Ingredients:
- 1 teaspoon olive oil
- 2 carrots, peeled and chopped
- 2 bell peppers, seeded and cut into strips
- ½ of eggplant, chopped
- 1 pound squids, cleaned
- 2 tablespoons fish sauce
- 1 teaspoon fresh ginger, minced
- ½ teaspoon paprika
- 1 cup fresh spinach, chopped

- Salt and ground black pepper, as needed
- 2 small zucchinis, spiralized with Blade C

Directions:
1. In a large-sized wok, heat oil over medium heat and stir fry carrots, bell pepper and eggplant for approximately 3-4 minutes.
2. Add in squids, fish sauce, ginger and paprika and cook for approximately 1-2 minutes.
3. Stir in spinach and cook for approximately 3-4 minutes.
4. Meanwhile, in a pan of boiling eater, add zucchini noodles and cook for approximately 1-2 minutes.
5. Drain the zucchini noodles well.
6. Transfer the zucchini noodles into 2 serving bowls.
7. Top with squid mixture and gently stir to blend.
8. Serve immediately.

Nutritional Information per Serving:
Calories: 177
Fat: 3.2g
Net Carbohydrates: 12.8g
Carbohydrates: 17.4g
Fiber: 4.6g
Sugar: 7.7g
Protein: 20.5g
Sodium: 819mg

CHAPTER 7:
Vegetarian Recipes

Broccoli Soup

Serves: 4 individuals
Preparation Time: 15 minutes
Cooking Time: 45 minutes

Ingredients:
- 1 tablespoon coconut oil
- 1 celery stalk, chopped
- ½ cup white onion, chopped
- Salt, as needed
- 1 teaspoon ground turmeric
- 2 garlic cloves, minced
- 1 large head broccoli, cut into florets
- ¼ teaspoon fresh ginger, grated
- 1 bay leaf
- 1/8 teaspoon cayenne powder
- Ground black pepper, as needed
- 5 cups homemade vegetable broth
- 1 small avocado, peeled, pitted and chopped
- 1 tablespoon fresh lemon juice

Directions:
1. In a large-sized soup pan, heat oil over medium heat and cook celery, onion and some salt for approximately 3-4 minutes.
2. Add turmeric and garlic and sauté for approximately 1 minute.
3. Add salt and remaining ingredients except for avocado and lemon juice and cook until boiling
4. Now, adjust the heat to medium-low and cook, covered for approximately 25-30 minutes.
5. Remove the pan of soup from heat and discard the bay leaf.
6. Set aside to cool slightly.
7. In a clean blender, add soup and avocado in batches and pulse until smooth.
8. Return the soup into the same pan over medium heat and cook for approximately 3-5 minutes.
9. Serve immediately with the drizzling of lemon juice.

Nutritional Information per Serving:
Calories: 169
Fat: 11g
Net Carbohydrates: 6.2g
Carbohydrates: 10.4g
Fiber: 4.2g
Sugar: 2.9g
Protein: 8.8g
Sodium: 709mg

Cauliflower Soup

Serves: 2 individuals
Preparation Time: 10 minutes
Cooking Time: 55 minutes

Ingredients:
- 2 teaspoons olive oil
- ½ cup onion, chopped
- 1 large head cauliflower, cut into small florets
- 1 (1-inch) piece fresh ginger, chopped
- Salt and ground black pepper, as needed
- 3 cups chicken bones broth

Directions:
1. In a large-sized soup pan, heat oil over medium heat and cook onion for approximately 1 minute.
2. Add cauliflower and cook, covered for approximately 10 minutes, stirring occasionally.
3. Add remaining ingredients and cook until boiling
4. Now, adjust the heat to low and cook, covered for approximately 30 minutes.
5. Remove the pan of soup from heat and set aside to cool slightly.
6. In a clean blender, add soup mixture in batches and pulse until smooth.
7. Return the soup in the pan over low heat and cook for approximately 4-5 minutes or until heated completely.
8. Serve immediately.

Nutritional Information per Serving:
Calories: 183
Fat: 6.2g
Net Carbohydrates: 16.9g
Carbohydrates: 28.4g
Fiber: 11.5g
Sugar: 12.6g
Protein: 9.8g
Sodium: 377mg

Pumpkin Soup

Serves: 4 individuals
Preparation Time: 15 minutes
Cooking Time: 25 minutes

Ingredients:
- 2 teaspoons coconut oil
- 1 brown onion, chopped
- 1 (¾-inch) fresh turmeric piece
- 1 (¾-inch) fresh galangal piece
- 1 long red chili, seeded and chopped
- 2 tablespoons fresh cilantro, chopped
- 4 kefir lime leaves
- 3 cups pumpkin, peeled and cubed
- 1 teaspoon fresh lime peel piece
- 1 large garlic clove, chopped
- 4 cups homemade vegetable broth
- 2 tablespoons red boat fish sauce
- ½ cup coconut cream
- 2 tablespoons fresh lime juice

Directions:
1. In a large-sized soup pan, heat oil over medium heat and cook onion, turmeric, galangal, red chili, cilantro and lime leaves for approximately 3-5 minutes.
2. Add pumpkin, lime peel, garlic, broth and fish sauce and cook until boiling
3. Now, adjust the heat to low and cook, covered for approximately 15 minutes.
4. Remove the pan of soup from heat and discard the turmeric, galangal and lemon peel.
5. Stir in the coconut cream and lemon juice and with an immersion blender, puree the soup until smooth.
6. Serve immediately.

Nutritional Information per Serving:
Calories: 189
Fat: 10.1g
Net Carbohydrates: 16.4g
Carbohydrates: 24.4g
Fiber: 8g
Sugar: 10.3g
Protein: 3.3g
Sodium: 546mg

Butternut Squash Soup

Serves: 6 individuals
Preparation Time: 15 minutes
Cooking Time: 40 minutes

Ingredients:
- 3 tablespoons olive oil
- 1 large onion, chopped finely
- 1 cup raw cashews
- 1 garlic clove, minced
- 2 tablespoons fresh ginger, minced
- 1 (2-pound) butternut squash, peeled and cubed into ½-inch size
- 2 teaspoons ground coriander
- 2 teaspoons ground cumin
- 1 teaspoon ground turmeric
- 1 teaspoon curry powder
- Salt and ground black pepper, as needed
- 5 cups homemade vegetable broth
- 1 cup unsweetened coconut milk

Directions:
1. In a large-sized soup pan, heat oil over medium heat and cook onion for approximately 5-6 minutes.
2. Add cashews and sauté for approximately 3 minutes.
3. Add garlic and ginger and sauté for approximately 1 minute.
4. Add remaining ingredients except for coconut milk and cook until boiling
5. Now, adjust the heat to low and cook, covered for approximately 20-25 minutes.
6. Remove the pan of soup from heat and stir in coconut milk.
7. With an immersion blender, puree the soup until smooth.
8. Serve immediately.

Nutritional Information per Serving:
Calories: 323
Fat: 18g
Net Carbohydrates: 33g
Carbohydrates: 39g
Fiber: 6g
Sugar: 7g
Protein: 7g
Sodium: 15mg

Carrot & Sweet Potato Soup

Serves: 5 individuals
Preparation Time: 15 minutes
Cooking Time: 45 minutes

Ingredients:
- 2 teaspoons olive oil
- ½ cup shallots, chopped
- 1½ cups carrots, peeled and sliced into ¼-inch size
- 3 cups sweet potato, peeled and cubed into ½-inch size
- 1 tablespoon fresh ginger, grated
- 2 teaspoons curry powder
- 3 cups chicken bones broth
- Salt and ground black pepper, as needed

Directions:

1. In a large-sized soup pan, heat oil over medium heat and sauté shallots for approximately 2-3 minutes.
2. Add carrot, sweet potato, ginger and curry powder and sauté for approximately 4-6 minutes.
3. Add broth and cook until boiling.
4. Now, adjust the heat to low and cook, covered for approximately 25-30 minutes.
5. Stir in salt and black pepper and remove from heat.
6. With an immersion blender, puree the soup until smooth.
7. Serve immediately.

Nutritional Information per Serving:

Calories: 131
Fat: 2.1g
Net Carbohydrates: 19.2g
Carbohydrates: 23.1g
Fiber: 3.9g
Sugar: 5.7g
Protein: 5.7g
Sodium: 539mg

Mixed Veggie Stew

Serves: 4 individuals
Preparation Time: 20 minutes
Cooking Time: 1 hour

Ingredients:

- 2 tablespoons olive oil
- 1¼ cups yellow onion, chopped
- 1 tablespoon garlic, minced
- 1 tablespoon chili paste
- 1½ tablespoons fresh turmeric, grated
- 1½ teaspoons ground cumin
- 1 teaspoon ground cinnamon
- 1 cup carrots, peeled and chopped roughly
- 1 cup cauliflower, chopped roughly
- 2 cups broccoli, chopped roughly
- 2 cups green cabbage, chopped roughly
- 1 cup coconut water
- 2 cups canned crushed tomatoes
- ¾ cup frozen green peas, thawed
- Salt and ground black pepper, as needed

Directions:

1. In a large-sized soup pan, heat oil over medium heat and cook onion and garlic for approximately 10 minutes, stirring occasionally.
2. Add chili paste, turmeric, cumin and cinnamon and sauté for approximately 1 minute.
3. Stir in carrots and cook for approximately 3-4 minutes.
4. Stir in cauliflower and broccoli and cook for approximately 2-3 minutes.

5. Stir in cabbage and immediately adjust the heat to low.
6. Cook for approximately 4-6 minutes.
7. Add coconut water and tomatoes and stir to blend.
8. Now, adjust the heat to high and cook until boiling.
9. Now, adjust the heat to low and cook, covered for approximately 30 minutes.
10. Stir in green peas, salt and black pepper and cook for approximately 3-5 minutes.
11. Serve hot.

Nutritional Information per Serving:

Calories: 216
Fat: 7.9g
Net Carbohydrates: 20.6g
Carbohydrates: 31.8g
Fiber: 11.2g
Sugar: 15.6g
Protein: 8.2g
Sodium: 395mg

Root Veggie & Kale Stew

Serves: 8 individuals
Preparation Time: 15 minutes
Cooking Time: 40 minutes

Ingredients:

- 2 tablespoons coconut oil
- 1 large sweet onion, chopped
- 1 medium parsnip, peeled and chopped
- 3 tablespoons tomato paste
- 4 garlic cloves, minced
- 1 teaspoon ground cumin
- ½ teaspoon ground cinnamon
- ½ teaspoon ground ginger
- ¼ teaspoon cayenne powder
- 2 medium carrots, peeled and chopped
- 2 medium purple potatoes, peeled and chopped
- 2 medium sweet potatoes, peeled and chopped
- 4 cups homemade vegetable broth
- 2 tablespoons fresh lemon juice
- 2 cups fresh kale, tough ribs removed and chopped roughly
- Salt and ground black pepper, as needed
- ¼ cup fresh cilantro leaves, chopped

Directions:

1. In a large-sized Dutch oven, melt the coconut oil over medium-high heat and sauté the onion for approximately 5 minutes.
2. Add the parsnip and sauté for approximately 3 minutes.
3. Stir in tomato paste, garlic and spices and sauté for approximately 2 minutes.
4. Add the carrots, potatoes and sweet potatoes and stir to blend.
5. Add the broth and cook until boiling.

6. Now, adjust the heat to medium-low and simmer for approximately 20 minutes.
7. Stir in the lemon juice and kale and simmer for approximately 4-5 minutes.
8. Stir in the salt and black pepper and serve hot with the garnishing of cilantro.

Nutritional Information per Serving:
Calories: 175
Fat: 4.5g
Net Carbohydrates: 23.5g
Carbohydrates: 29g
Fiber: 5.5g
Sugar: 5.2g
Protein: 5.8g
Sodium: 429mg

Tofu & Veggie Stew
Serves: 6 individuals
Preparation Time: 15 minutes
Cooking Time: 30 minutes

Ingredients:
- 2 tablespoons garlic, peeled
- 1 tablespoon fresh ginger, peeled
- 1 jalapeño pepper, seeded and chopped
- 1 (16-ounce) jar roasted red peppers, rinsed, drained and chopped
- 2 cups homemade vegetable broth
- 2 cups water
- 1 medium red bell pepper, seeded and thinly sliced
- 1 small zucchini, sliced
- 1 (16-ounce) package extra-firm tofu, drained and cubed
- 1 (10-ounce) package frozen spinach, thawed

Directions:
1. In a clean food processor, place the garlic, jalapeño pepper and roasted red peppers and pulse until smooth.
2. In a large-sized saucepan, add the peppers puree, broth, and water over medium-high heat and cook until boiling.
3. Add the bell pepper, zucchini and tofu and stir to blend.
4. Now, adjust the heat to medium and cook for approximately 5 minutes.
5. Stir in the spinach and cook for approximately 5 minutes.
6. Serve hot.

Nutritional Information per Serving:
Calories: 126
Fat: 5.3g
Net Carbohydrates: 8.5g
Carbohydrates: 11.4g

Fiber: 2.9g
Sugar: 5.6g
Protein: 11.8g
Sodium: 483mg

Banana & Tomato Curry
Serves: 4 individuals
Preparation Time: 15 minutes
Cooking Time: 17 minutes

Ingredients:
- 2 tablespoons olive oil
- 2 onions, chopped
- 8 garlic cloves, minced
- 1 teaspoon coconut sugar
- 1 tablespoon curry powder
- ½ teaspoon ground ginger
- ½ teaspoon ground cumin
- ½ teaspoon ground turmeric
- ½ teaspoon ground cinnamon
- 1 teaspoon red chili powder
- Salt and ground black pepper, as needed
- 2/3 cup fat-free plain Greek yogurt
- 1 (10-ounce) can sugar-free tomato sauce
- 2 large bananas, peeled and sliced
- 3 tomatoes, chopped
- ¼ cup unsweetened coconut flakes

Directions:
1. In a large-sized saucepan, heat oil over medium heat and cook onion for approximately 4-5 minutes.
2. Add garlic, curry powder, sugar and spices and sauté for approximately 1 minute.
3. Add yogurt and tomato sauce and bring to a gentle boil.
4. Stir in bananas and simmer for approximately 3 minutes.
5. Stir in tomatoes and simmer for approximately 1-2 minutes.
6. Stir in coconut flakes and immediately remove from heat.
7. Serve hot.

Nutritional Information per Serving:
Calories: 290
Fat: 15.6g
Net Carbohydrates: 27.5g
Carbohydrates: 35.4g
Fiber: 7.9g
Sugar: 16.8g
Protein: 6.2g
Sodium: 450mg

Potato Curry

Serves: 4 individuals
Preparation Time: 10 minutes
Cooking Time: 25 minutes

Ingredients:

- 1 pound potatoes, peeled and cubed into 1½-inh size
- 2 garlic cloves, minced
- 1 teaspoon fresh ginger, minced
- 4 fresh curry leaves
- 2 teaspoons curry powder
- ½ teaspoon cayenne powder
- 1½-2 cups coconut cream
- 1 cup water
- 2 tablespoons fresh cilantro, chopped

Directions:

1. In a large-sized-heavy-bottomed saucepan, blend together potato and remaining ingredients except for cilantro.
2. Place the pan of potato mixture over medium heat and cook for approximately 20-25 minutes, stirring occasionally.
3. Discard the curry leaves and serve hot with the garnishing of cilantro.

Nutritional Information per Serving:

Calories: 293
Fat: 21.8g
Net Carbohydrates: 19.2g
Carbohydrates: 24.4g
Fiber: 5.2g
Sugar: 4.4g
Protein: 4.3g
Sodium: 23mg

Pumpkin Curry

Serves: 4 individuals
Preparation Time: 15 minutes
Cooking Time: 30 minutes

Ingredients:
For Roasted Pumpkin:
- 1 medium sugar pumpkin, peeled and cubed
- Salt and ground black pepper, as needed
- 1 teaspoon olive oil

For Curry:
- 1 teaspoon olive oil
- 1 onion, chopped
- 1 tablespoon fresh ginger, minced
- 1 tablespoon garlic, minced
- 1½ cups canned sugar-free pumpkin puree
- 1 cup unsweetened coconut milk
- 2 cups homemade vegetable broth
- 1 tablespoon curry powder
- 1 teaspoon smoked paprika
- 1 teaspoon ground cumin
- 12 teaspoon ground turmeric
- Salt, as needed
- 10 curry leaves
- 1 tablespoon fresh lime juice
- 2 tablespoons fresh parsley, chopped

Directions:
1. Preheat your oven to 400 °F.
2. Line a large-sized baking sheet with parchment paper.
3. For roasted pumpkin: in a large-sized bowl, add all ingredients and toss to combine.
4. Place pumpkin cubes onto the prepared baking sheet and then arrange in a single layer.
5. Roast for approximately 20-25 minutes, flipping once halfway through.
6. Meanwhile for curry: in a large-sized saucepan, heat oil over medium-high heat and cook onion for approximately 4-5 minutes.
7. Add ginger and garlic and sauté for approximately 1 minute.
8. Stir in pumpkin puree and immediately adjust the heat to medium-low.
9. Cook for approximately 10 minutes, stirring occasionally.
10. Add in coconut milk, broth, spices and curry leaves and cook until boiling.
11. Now, adjust the heat to low and cook for approximately 15 minutes.
12. Stir in roasted pumpkin and simmer for 3-5 minutes more.
13. Serve hot with the garnishing of parsley.

Nutritional Information per Serving:
Calories: 255
Fat: 12.9g
Net Carbohydrates: 20.1g
Carbohydrates: 29.6g
Fiber: 9.5g
Sugar: 10.5g
Protein: 6.9g
Sodium: 457mg

Mushrooms & Corn Curry

Serves: 4 individuals
Preparation Time: 15 minutes
Cooking Time: 20 minutes

Ingredients:
- 2 cups tomatoes, chopped
- 1 green chili, chopped
- 1 teaspoon fresh ginger, chopped
- ¼ cup cashews
- 2 tablespoons olive oil
- ½ teaspoon cumin seeds
- ¼ teaspoon ground coriander
- ¼ teaspoon ground turmeric
- ¼ teaspoon red chili powder
- 1½ cups fresh shiitake mushrooms, sliced
- 1½ cups fresh button mushrooms, sliced
- 1 cup frozen corn kernels
- 1¼ cups water
- ¼ cup unsweetened coconut milk
- Salt and ground black pepper, as needed

Directions:
1. In a clean food processor, add tomatoes, green chili, ginger and cashews and pulse until a smooth paste forms.
2. In a large-sized saucepan, heat oil over medium heat and sauté cumin seeds for approximately 1 minute.
3. Add spices and sauté for approximately 1 minute.
4. Add tomato paste and cook for approximately 5 minutes.
5. Stir in mushrooms, corn, water, coconut milk, salt and black pepper and cook for approximately 10-12 minutes, stirring occasionally.
6. Serve hot.

Nutritional Information per Serving:
Calories: 208
Fat: 15.3g
Net Carbohydrates: 14g
Carbohydrates: 17.4g
Fiber: 3.4g
Sugar: 5.5g
Protein: 5.3g
Sodium: 55mg

Asparagus & Spinach Curry

Serves: 4 individuals
Preparation Time: 15 minutes
Cooking Time: 20 minutes

Ingredients:

- 2 teaspoons coconut oil
- 1 small white onion, chopped
- 2 garlic cloves, chopped finely
- 1 tablespoon fresh ginger, chopped finely
- Salt, as needed
- 3 carrots, peeled and cut into ¾-inch round slices
- 2 cups asparagus, trimmed and cut into 2-inch pieces
- 2 tablespoons green curry paste
- 1½ teaspoons coconut sugar
- 1 (14-ounce) can unsweetened coconut milk
- ½ cup water
- 2 cups fresh baby spinach, chopped roughly
- 1½ teaspoons coconut aminos
- 1½ teaspoons balsamic vinegar
- ½ teaspoon red pepper flakes

Directions:

1. In a large-sized deep wok, melt coconut oil over medium heat and cook the onion, garlic, ginger and a pinch of salt for approximately 5 minutes.
2. Add carrots and asparagus and cook for approximately 3-4 minutes, stirring occasionally.
3. Stir in the curry paste and cook for approximately 2 minutes, stirring occasionally.
4. Add coconut sugar, coconut milk and water and bring to a gentle simmer.
5. Cook for approximately 6-10 minutes or until desired doneness of vegetables.
6. Stir in the spinach and cook for approximately 2-3 minutes.
7. Stir in coconut aminos, vinegar, salt and red pepper flakes and remove from heat.
8. Serve hot.

Nutritional Information per Serving:

Calories: 249
Fat: 17.7g
Net Carbohydrates: 14g
Carbohydrates: 17.5g
Fiber: 3.5g
Sugar: 8.4g
Protein: 4g
Sodium: 419mg

Veggies & Pumpkin Puree Curry

Serves: 4 individuals
Preparation Time: 15 minutes
Cooking Time: 35 minutes

Ingredients:

- 1 tablespoon coconut oil
- 1 green bell pepper, seeded and chopped
- 1 onion, chopped
- 1 cup sugar-free pumpkin puree
- 1 sweet potato, peeled and cut into 1-inch cubes
- 1 head broccoli, cut into florets
- 1 tablespoon curry powder
- 1 teaspoon ground cinnamon
- ¼ teaspoon ground ginger
- Salt, as needed
- 1 (14-ounce) can unsweetened coconut milk
- 1 cup water

Directions:

1. In a large-sized saucepan, melt coconut oil over medium heat and cook onion for approximately 8-10 minutes.
2. Add in pumpkin puree and remaining ingredients and stir to blend.
3. Now, adjust the heat to high and cook until boiling.
4. Now, adjust the heat to low and cook, covered for approximately 15-20 minutes.
5. Serve hot.

Nutritional Information per Serving:

Calories: 280
Fat: 17.8g
Net Carbohydrates: 18.8g
Carbohydrates: 25.2g
Fiber: 6.4g
Sugar: 10.6g
Protein: 5.2g
Sodium: 111mg

Tofu & Veggie Curry

Serves: 6 individuals
Preparation Time: 15 minutes
Cooking Time: 35 minutes

Ingredients:

- 2 tablespoons olive oil
- ½ cup shallots, chopped finely
- 4 garlic cloves, minced
- 2 tablespoons fresh ginger, minced
- ¼ cup peanut butter
- 1 teaspoon hot chili paste
- 1 teaspoon curry powder
- 1 teaspoon ground cumin

- 1 teaspoon ground turmeric
- 1 (14-ounce) can unsweetened coconut milk
- 1¼ cups water
- 1 tablespoon coconut sugar
- 3 fresh lime leaves
- 2 (14-ounce) packages firm tofu, pressed, drained and cubed into 1-inch size
- 2 large bell peppers, seeded and cut into ¾-inch pieces
- 3 medium carrots, peeled and cut into ¼-inch slices
- Salt and ground black pepper, as needed

Directions:
1. In a large-sized saucepan, heat oil over medium-high heat and sauté shallot, garlic and ginger for approximately 3-4 minutes.
2. Add peanut butter, chili paste and spices and cook, stirring for approximately 1 minute.
3. Add coconut milk, water, coconut sugar and lime leaves and cook until boiling.
4. Add in tofu and remaining ingredients and again cook until boiling.
5. Now, adjust the heat to medium-low and cook for approximately 20 minutes, stirring occasionally.
6. Serve hot.

Nutritional Information per Serving:
Calories: 353
Fat: 25.2g
Net Carbohydrates: 15.5g
Carbohydrates: 19.1g
Fiber: 3.6g
Sugar: 9.3g
Protein: 15.8g
Sodium: 150mg

Spicy Veggie Curry
Serves: 6 individuals
Preparation Time: 20 minutes
Cooking Time: 40 minutes

Ingredients:
- 2 tablespoons olive oil
- 1 teaspoon mustard seeds
- 2 onions, chopped finely
- 2 fresh green chilies, seeded and chopped
- 1 bunch curry leaves
- ½ teaspoon garam masala
- ½ teaspoon ground cumin
- ½ teaspoon ground coriander
- ¼ teaspoon ground turmeric
- ¼ teaspoon red chili powder
- 6 tomatoes, chopped
- 1 eggplant, cubed

- 2 potatoes, peeled and cubed
- 2 sweet potatoes, peeled and cubed
- ½ cup unsweetened coconut milk
- ½ cup okra, trimmed and chopped
- ½ cup French beans
- ½ cup fresh green peas, shelled
- Salt and ground black pepper, as needed

Directions:
1. In a large-sized saucepan, heat oil over medium heat and sauté mustard seeds for approximately 1 minute.
2. Add onion, green chilies, curry leaves and spices and sauté for approximately 4-5 minutes.
3. Add tomatoes and cook for approximately 2-3 minutes.
4. Stir in eggplant, potatoes, sweet potatoes and coconut milk and bring to a gentle simmer.
5. Now, adjust the heat to medium-low and cook, covered for approximately 15-20 minutes or until desired doneness.
6. Stir in the okra, French beans, green peas, salt and black pepper and cook for approximately 5 minutes.
7. Serve hot.

Nutritional Information per Serving:
Calories: 300
Fat: 8.6g
Net Carbohydrates: 36.4g
Carbohydrates: 49.9g
Fiber: 13.5g
Sugar: 9.5g
Protein: 8.3g
Sodium: 57mg

Stuffed Zucchini
Serves: 8 individuals
Preparation Time: 20 minutes
Cooking Time: 30 minutes

Ingredients:
- 4 medium zucchinis, halved lengthwise
- Salt, as needed
- 1½ baking potatoes, peeled and cubed
- 4 teaspoons olive oil
- 2½ cups onion, chopped
- 1 Serrano chili, mined
- 2 garlic cloves, minced
- 1½ tablespoons fresh ginger, minced
- 2 tablespoons chickpea flour
- 1 teaspoon ground coriander
- ¼ teaspoon ground cumin
- ¼ teaspoon ground turmeric
- Ground black pepper, as needed

- 1½ cups frozen green peas, thawed
- 2 tablespoons fresh cilantro, chopped

Directions:
1. Preheat your oven to 375 °F.
2. With a scooper, scoop out the pulp from zucchini halves, leaving about ¼-inch thick shell.
3. In a shallow roasting pan, arrange the zucchini halves, cut side up.
4. Sprinkle the zucchini halves with a little salt.
5. In a saucepan of boiling water, cook the potatoes for approximately 2 minutes.
6. Drain the potatoes well and set aside.
7. In a large-sized non-stick wok, heat oil over medium-high heat and cook onion, Serrano, garlic and ginger for approximately 3 minutes.
8. Now, adjust the heat to medium-low and stir in chickpea flour and spices.
9. Cook for approximately 5 minutes, stirring continuously.
10. Sir in cooked potato, green peas and cilantro and remove the wok from heat.
11. With a paper towel, pat dry the zucchini halves.
12. Stuff the zucchini halves with the veggie mixture evenly.
13. Cover the baking dish and bake for approximately 20 minutes.
14. Serve hot.

Nutritional Information per Serving
Calories: 169
Fat: 3.2g
Net Carbohydrates: 24.5g
Carbohydrates: 32.1g
Fiber: 7.6g
Sugar: 11.3g
Protein: 6.5g
Sodium: 260mg

Veggie Gumbo

Serves: 6 individuals
Preparation Time: 15 minutes
Cooking Time: 55 minutes

Ingredients:
- 3 tablespoon olive oil, divided
- 1 medium bell pepper, seeded and chopped finely
- 1 medium onion, chopped finely
- 1 garlic clove, minced
- 1 teaspoon fresh ginger, minced
- 8 ounces fresh mushrooms, sliced
- ½ of (16-ounce) package frozen okra, thawed, trimmed and sliced
- 1 (14½-ounce) can diced tomatoes with liquid
- 1 (6-ounce) can sugar-free tomato paste
- 2 bay leaves
- 1 teaspoon dried thyme, crushed
- ½ teaspoon cayenne powder
- ¼ teaspoon red pepper flakes, crushed
- Salt and ground black pepper, as needed

- 2 tablespoons almond flour

Directions:
1. In a large-sized saucepan, heat 1 tablespoon of oil over medium heat and cook bell pepper, onion and garlic and sauté for approximately 4-5 minutes.
2. Stir in mushrooms, okra, tomatoes, tomato paste, bay leaves, thyme and spices and cook for approximately 40 minutes, stirring occasionally.
3. Meanwhile, in a frying pan, heat remaining oil over medium heat.
4. Gradually add flour, stirring continuously until smooth.
5. Cook for approximately 3-5 minutes or until a golden brown roux forms, , stirring continuously.
6. Add the roux in gumbo mixture, stirring continuously.
7. Cook for approximately 5-10 minutes or until thickens, stirring occasionally.
8. Serve hot.

Nutritional Information per Serving:
Calories: 177
Fat: 11g
Net Carbohydrates: 12.3g
Carbohydrates: 17.4g
Fiber: 5.1g
Sugar: 8.4g
Protein: 5.7g
Sodium: 39mg

Nutty Veggie Combo

Serves: 12 individuals
Preparation Time: 20 minutes
Cooking Time: 1 hour 1 minute

Ingredients:

- 1½ cups pecans
- 1 small butternut squash, peeled, seeded and cut into ¼-thick slices
- 1 medium head cauliflower, cut into florets
- 1 pound Brussels sprouts, trimmed and halved
- 2 large parsnips, peeled and cut into ¼-thick slices
- 4 medium carrots, peeled and cut into ¼-thick slices
- ¼ teaspoon nutmeg, grated freshly
- Salt and ground black pepper, as needed
- ½ cup extra-virgin olive oil
- 2 tablespoons fresh ginger, minced
- 1/3 cup organic honey

Directions:

1. Preheat your oven to 425 °F.
2. In a pie plate, place the pecans and roast for approximately 6 minutes or until toasted.
3. Meanwhile, in a large-sized bowl, add all vegetables, nutmeg, salt, black pepper and oil and toss to combine.
4. Divide the vegetable mixture onto 2 large rimmed baking sheets and then spread in an even layer.
5. Remove the pecans from oven and set aside.
6. Again, set the temperature of your oven to 425 °F.
7. Place the baking sheets of vegetables into the oven and roast for approximately 55 minutes.
8. After 30 minutes of cooking, sprinkle the top of vegetables with ginger and pecans.
9. Then drizzle with honey evenly.
10. Serve hot.

Nutritional Information per Serving:

Calories: 293
Fat: 20.1g
Net Carbohydrates: 22.9g
Carbohydrates: 29.7g
Fiber: 6.8g
Sugar: 13.3g
Protein: 4.7g
Sodium: 147mg

Tempeh in Tomato Sauce

Serves: 4 individuals
Preparation Time: 15 minutes
Cooking Time: 1½ hours

Ingredients:

- 1/3 cup olive oil, divided
- 2 (8-ounce) packages tempeh, cut into ½-inch slices horizontally
- 1 large onion, chopped
- 3 garlic cloves, minced
- 1 teaspoon dried oregano, crushed
- 1 teaspoon dried thyme, crushed
- 1 teaspoon red chili powder
- 1 teaspoon paprika
- ½ teaspoon red pepper flakes, crushed
- 2 large green bell peppers, seeded and sliced thinly
- 1 (14½-ounce) can diced tomatoes
- ¼ cup canned sugar-free tomato paste
- 1 teaspoon balsamic vinegar
- 1 tablespoon maple syrup

Directions:

1. Preheat your oven to 350 °F.
2. In a large-sized bowl, add 2 tablespoons of oil and tempeh slices and toss to combine.
3. In a large-sized, non-stick wok, heat 2 tablespoons of oil over medium-high heat and cook the tempeh slices for approximately 5-7 minutes.
4. Carefully change the side and cook for approximately 5-7 minutes.
5. Transfer the cooked tempeh slices onto a paper towel-lined plate. Keep aside.
6. Meanwhile in another non-stick wok, heat remaining oil over medium-low heat and cook onion, garlic, herbs and spices for approximately 8-10 minutes.
7. Add bell pepper and cook for approximately 4-5 minutes.
8. Add tomatoes, tomato paste, vinegar and maple syrup and stir until blended thoroughly.
9. Transfer the tempeh slices into a large-sized casserole dish.
10. Place tomato mixture over tempeh slices evenly.
11. With a piece of foil, cover the casserole dish and bake for approximately 1 hour.
12. Serve hot.

Nutritional Information per Serving:

Calories: 449
Fat: 29.8g
Net Carbohydrates: 25.4g
Carbohydrates: 30.3g
Fiber: 4.9g
Sugar: 11.4g
Protein: 24.1g
Sodium: 43mg

CHAPTER 8:
Wraps & Sandwiches Recipes

Zucchini Lettuce Wraps

Serves: 4 individuals
Preparation Time: 15 minutes
Cooking Time: 14 minutes

Ingredients:
- 1 tablespoon olive oil
- 1 teaspoon cumin seeds
- 1 small yellow onion, sliced thinly
- 4 cups zucchini, grated
- ½ teaspoon red pepper flakes, crushed
- Salt and ground black pepper, as needed
- 8 large lettuce leaves, rinsed and pat dried
- 2 tablespoons fresh chives, minced finely

Directions:
1. In a medium-sized wok, heat the oil over medium-high heat and sauté the cumin seeds for approximately 1 minute.
2. Add the onion and sauté for approximately 4-5 minutes.
3. Add the zucchini and cook for approximately 5-7 minutes or until done completely, stirring occasionally.
4. Stir in the red pepper flakes, salt and black pepper and remove from the heat.
5. Arrange the lettuce leaves onto a smooth surface.
6. Divide the zucchini mixture onto each lettuce leaf evenly.
7. Top with the chives and serve immediately.

Nutritional Information per Serving:
Calories: 60
Fat: 3.9g
Net Carbohydrates: 4.4g
Carbohydrates: 6.2g
Fiber: 1.8g
Sugar: 2.9g
Protein: 1.8g
Sodium: 52mg

Veggie Lettuce Wraps

Serves: 3 individuals
Preparation Time: 14 minutes

Ingredients:
- ¾ cup fresh kale, tough ribs removed and torn
- 1 cup cucumber, sliced
- 1 cup cherry tomatoes, halved
- 1 tablespoon fresh lemon juice
- ¼ teaspoon ground ginger
- ¼ teaspoon ground cumin
- Salt, as needed
- 6 large lettuce leaves

Directions:
1. In a large-sized bowl, add the kale, cucumber, tomatoes, lemon juice, spices and salt and mix well.

2. Arrange the lettuce leaves onto serving plates.
3. Divide the kale mixture onto each lettuce leaf evenly.
4. Serve immediately.

Nutritional Information per Serving:
Calories: 28
Fat: 0.3g
Net Carbohydrates: 4.6g
Carbohydrates: 5.9g
Fiber: 1.3g
Sugar: 2.4g
Protein: 1.4g
Sodium: 63mg

Chickpeas Lettuce Wraps

Serves: 4 individuals
Preparation Time: 15 minutes
Cooking Time: 25 minutes

Ingredients:
- 1 (16-ounce) can chickpeas, drained, rinsed and pat dried
- 2 tablespoons olive oil
- ½ teaspoon garlic powder
- ¼ teaspoon paprika
- ¼ teaspoon ground cumin
- 8 large lettuce leaves
- 1 avocado, peeled, pitted and chopped
- 2 cups cherry tomatoes, halved

Directions:
1. Preheat your oven to 400 °F.
2. Line a large-sized baking sheet with parchment paper.
3. In a bowl, add the chickpeas, oil, spices and salt and toss to combine.
4. Place the chickpeas onto the prepared baking sheet and then spread in an even layer.
5. Bake for approximately 20-25 minutes or until crispy.
6. Transfer the chickpeas into a glass bowl and set aside to cool.
7. Arrange the lettuce leaves onto serving plates.
8. Divide the chickpeas, avocado and tomatoes over each leaf evenly.
9. Serve immediately.

Nutritional Information per Serving
Calories: 317
Fat: 18.3g
Net Carbohydrates: 24.5g
Carbohydrates: 34.1g
Fiber: 9.6g
Sugar: 2.8g
Protein: 7.5g
Sodium: 347mg

Beans & Rice Lettuce Wraps

Serves: 5 individuals
Preparation Time: 15 minutes

Ingredients:

- 1 (15-ounce) can black beans, drained
- ½ cup cooked brown rice
- ½ cup low-fat feta cheese, crumbled
- ½ cup scallion, chopped
- 1 garlic clove, minced
- ¼ teaspoon fresh ginger, minced
- 2 tablespoons fresh lemon juice
- Salt and ground black pepper, as needed
- 10 Boston lettuce leaves

Directions:

1. Place all the ingredients except lettuce leaves in a bowl and mix well.
2. Place 2 lettuce leaves onto each serving plate.
3. Place beans mixture over each leaf evenly.
4. Serve immediately.

Nutritional Information per Serving:

Calories: 163
Fat: 2.1g
Net Carbohydrates: 18g
Carbohydrates: 26.3g
Fiber: 8.3g
Sugar: 0.5g
Protein: 10.7g
Sodium: 91mg

Beans & Veggies Lettuce Wraps

Serves: 5 individuals
Preparation Time: 15 minutes

Ingredients:
For Dressing:

- 2 tablespoons fresh cilantro leaves, chopped
- 1 tablespoon shallots, minced
- 1 teaspoon fresh lime zest, grated
- 1 tablespoon Dijon mustard
- 2½ tablespoons extra-virgin olive oil
- 2 tablespoons fresh lime juice
- 1 tablespoon apple cider vinegar
- Salt and ground black pepper, as needed

For Wraps:

- 1 (15-ounce) can white beans, drained
- 1 cup fresh cucumber, chopped
- 1 cup carrot, peeled and chopped
- 1 large avocado, peeled, pitted and chopped
- 10 lettuce leaves

Directions:

1. For dressing: place the ingredients in a glass bowl and whisk until blended thoroughly.
2. Add the chickpeas, cucumber and carrot and mix well.

3. Gently, fold in the avocado.
4. Place the lettuce leaves onto serving plates.
5. Divide the chickpeas mixture over each leaf evenly and serve.

Nutritional Information per Serving:

Calories: 267
Fat: 14.3g
Net Carbohydrates: 16.8g
Carbohydrates: 28.9g
Fiber: 12.1g
Sugar: 2.1g
Protein: 8.2g
Sodium: 287mg

Quinoa Lettuce Wraps

Serves: 4 individuals
Preparation Time: 15 minutes
Cooking Time: 10 minutes

Ingredients:
For Filling:

- 1 teaspoon olive oil
- 2 cups fresh shiitake mushrooms, chopped
- 1 cup cooked quinoa
- 1 teaspoon fresh lime juice
- 1 teaspoon balsamic vinegar
- ¼ cup scallion, chopped
- Pinch of salt
- Ground black pepper, as needed

For Wraps:

- 8 medium butter lettuce leaves
- ¼ cup cucumber, peeled and julienned
- ¼ cup carrot, peeled and julienned
- 2 tablespoons unsalted peanuts, chopped

Directions:

1. For filling in a wok, heat oil over medium heat and cook the mushrooms for approximately 5-8 minutes.
2. Stir on quinoa, lime juice and vinegar and cook for approximately 1 minute.
3. Stir in scallion, salt and black pepper and immediately, remove from heat.
4. Let it cool.
5. Place lettuce leaves into serving plates.
6. Place quinoa filling over each leaf evenly.
7. Top with cucumber, carrot and peanuts and serve.

Nutritional Information per Serving:

Calories: 176
Fat: 5.4g
Net Carbohydrates: 21.9g
Carbohydrates: 25.8g
Fiber: 3.9g
Sugar: 2.4g

Protein: 7.2g
Sodium: 18mg

Chicken & Strawberry Lettuce Wraps

Serves: 4 individuals
Preparation Time: 15 minutes

Ingredients:
- 4 ounces cooked chicken, cut into strips
- ½ cup fresh strawberries, hulled and thinly sliced
- 1 small cucumber, thinly sliced
- 1 tablespoon fresh mint leaves, chopped
- 4 large lettuce leaves

Directions:
1. In a large-sized bowl, add all ingredients except for lettuce leaves and gently toss to combine.
2. Place the lettuce leaves onto serving plates.
3. Divide the chicken mixture over each leaf evenly.
4. Serve immediately.

Nutritional Information per Serving:
Calories: 122
Fat: 2g
Net Carbohydrates: 7.1g
Carbohydrates: 8.8g
Fiber: 1.7g
Sugar: 4.4g
Protein: 17.8g
Sodium: 41mg

Turkey Lettuce Wraps

Serves: 4 individuals
Preparation Time: 15 minutes
Cooking Time: 20 minutes

Ingredients:
- 1 tablespoon olive oil
- 1 cup onion, chopped
- ¾ pound extra-lean ground turkey
- 1 cup fresh mushrooms, chopped
- ½ tablespoon fresh ginger, minced
- ½ tablespoon cayenne powder
- ½ tablespoon ground cumin
- 8 large romaine lettuce leaves
- 2 tablespoons fresh cilantro leaves, chopped

Directions:
1. In a non-stick wok, heat oil over medium heat and cook the onion for approximately 4-5 minutes, stirring frequently.
2. Add turkey and cook, stirring occasionally for approximately 6-8 minutes.
3. Add mushrooms, ginger, cayenne powder and cumin and cook for approximately 5-7 minutes.
4. Remove the wok of turkey mixture from heat and set aside.
5. Arrange the lettuce leaves onto serving plates.
6. Place turkey mixture over each lettuce leaf evenly.
7. Top with cilantro evenly and serve.

Nutritional Information per Serving:
Calories: 236
Fat: 16.8g
Net Carbohydrates: 3.6g
Carbohydrates: 4.8g
Fiber: 1.2g
Sugar: 1.7g
Protein: 16.4g
Sodium: 58mg

Shrimp Lettuce Wraps

Serves: 4 individuals
Preparation Time: 15 minutes
Cooking Time: 5 minutes

Ingredients:
- 2 teaspoons olive oil
- 1 garlic clove, minced
- 1½ pounds shrimp, peeled, deveined and chopped
- Salt, as needed
- 8 large lettuce leaves
- ½ cup carrot, peeled and julienned
- ½ cup cucumber, julienned
- 2 tablespoons fresh lime juice
- 4 tablespoons fresh parsley, finely chopped

Directions:
1. Heat the olive oil in a large-sized wok over medium heat and sauté garlic for approximately 1 minute.
2. Add the shrimp and cook for approximately 3-4 minutes.
3. Remove the wok of shrimp from heat and set aside to cool slightly.
4. Arrange lettuce leaves onto serving plates.
5. Divide the shrimp, carrot and cucumber over the leaves evenly and drizzle with lime juice
6. Garnish with parsley and serve immediately.

Nutritional Information per Serving
Calories: 241
Fat: 5.3g
Net Carbohydrates: 5.4g
Carbohydrates: 6g
Fiber: 0.6g
Sugar: 1g
Protein: 39.1g
Sodium: 466mg

Veggie Tortilla Wraps

Serves: 4 individuals
Preparation Time: 15 minutes
Cooking Time: 22 minutes
Ingredients:

- 1½ cups broccoli florets, chopped
- 1½ cups cauliflower florets, chopped
- 1 tablespoon water
- 2 teaspoons olive oil
- 1½ cups onion, chopped
- 1 garlic clove, minced
- 2 tablespoons fresh parsley, finely chopped
- 4 eggs, beaten
- Salt and ground black pepper, as needed
- 4 whole-wheat tortillas, warmed

Instructions:

1. In a microwave-safe bowl, place broccoli, cauliflower and water and microwave, covered for approximately 3-5 minutes.
2. Remove from microwave and drain any liquid.
3. Heat olive oil in a wok over medium heat and sauté onion for approximately 4-5 minutes.
4. Add garlic and sauté for approximately 1 minute.
5. Stir in broccoli, cauliflower, parsley, eggs, salt and black pepper.
6. Now, Now, adjust the heat to medium-low and simmer for approximately 10 minutes.
7. Remove the wok of veggies from heat and set it aside to cool slightly.
8. Place broccoli mixture over ¼ of each tortilla.
9. Fold the outside edges inward and roll up like a burrito.
10. Secure the tortilla with toothpicks to secure the filling.
11. Cut each tortilla in half and serve.

Nutritional Information per Serving:
Calories: 147
Fat: 3.2g
Net Carbohydrates: 15.4g
Carbohydrates: 19.8g
Fiber: 4.4g
Sugar: 4g
Protein: 11.2g
Sodium: 156mg

Chicken & Mango Tortilla Wraps

Serves: 4 individuals
Preparation Time: 15 minutes

Ingredients:

- 2 tablespoons fresh lime juice
- 2 tablespoons olive oil
- 1 tablespoon Dijon mustard
- Ground black pepper, as needed
- 2 cups cooked chicken meat, shredded
- 1 cup mango, peeled, pitted and cut into cubes
- 1 cup purple cabbage, shredded
- ¼ cup fresh cilantro, chopped
- 4 (10-inch) whole-wheat tortillas, warmed
- 2 tablespoons fresh lime juice
- 2 tablespoons olive oil
- 1 tablespoon Dijon mustard
- Ground black pepper, as needed
- 2 cups cooked chicken meat, shredded
- 1 cup mango, peeled, pitted and cut into cubes
- 1 cup purple cabbage, shredded
- ¼ cup fresh cilantro, chopped
- 4 whole-wheat tortillas, warmed

Directions:

1. In a large-sized bowl, add mustard, lime juice, oil and black pepper and whisk until blended thoroughly.
2. Add beef, mango, cabbage and cilantro and toss to combine.
3. Arrange the tortillas onto a smooth surface.
4. Place beef mixture over each tortilla, leaving about 1-inch border all around.
5. Carefully fold the edges of each tortilla over the filling to roll up.
6. Cut each roll in half cross-wise and serve.

Nutritional Information per Serving
Calories: 296
Fat: 13.1g
Net Carbohydrates: 15.5g
Carbohydrates: 18.3g
Fiber: 2.8g
Sugar: 6.4g
Protein: 26.8g
Sodium: 113mg

Chicken & Tomato Tortilla Wraps

Serves: 6 individuals
Preparation Time: 16 minutes
Cooking Time: 7 minutes

Ingredients:

- 1 teaspoon olive oil
- 4 (4-ounce) boneless, skinless chicken breasts, cubed
- 1 cup onion, chopped
- 1 teaspoon fresh ginger, minced
- 1 garlic clove, minced
- Salt and ground black pepper, as needed
- 1 cup fresh tomato, chopped
- 1 cup fresh cilantro, chopped
- ½ cup salsa
- 6 (8-inch) whole-wheat tortillas

Directions:

1. In a large-sized, non-stick saucepan, heat oil and cook chicken, onion, ginger, garlic, salt and black pepper for approximately 5-7 minutes, stirring frequently.
2. Remove the wok of chicken from heat and stir in tomatoes, cilantro and salsa.
3. Place the tortillas onto plates and coat the outside edge of each with water.
4. Place about ½ cup of chicken mixture on each tortilla, leaving about ½-inch around the outer rim.
5. Place the chicken mixture over ¼ of each tortilla.
6. Fold the outside edges inward and roll up like a burrito.
7. Secure the tortilla with toothpicks to secure the filling.
8. Cut each tortilla in half and serve.

Nutritional Information per Serving:

Calories: 233
Fat: 7.1g
Net Carbohydrates: 13.4g
Carbohydrates: 15.8g
Fiber: 2.4g
Sugar: 3.2g
Protein: 25.1g
Sodium: 134mg

Banana Sandwiches

Serves: 2 individuals
Preparation Time: 10 minutes
Cooking Time: 6 minutes

Ingredients:

- Olive oil cooking spray
- 4 whole-wheat breads slices, toasted
- 4 teaspoons smooth peanut butter
- 2 ripe bananas, peeled and sliced

Directions:

1. Grease a grill pan with cooking spray and heat over medium heat.
2. Spread the peanut butter over 1 side of both bread slices.
3. Place banana slices over the buttered side of 1 slice.
4. Cover with the remaining slice and press firmly.
5. Cook the sandwich over grill pan for approximately 3 minutes per side.
6. Cut the sandwiches in half and serve.

Nutritional Information per Serving:

Calories: 281
Fat: 8.2g
Net Carbohydrates: 43.1g
Carbohydrates: 50g
Fiber: 6.9g
Sugar: 17g
Protein: 10.4g
Sodium: 245mg

Avocado & Tomato Sandwiches

Serves: 4 individuals
Preparation Time: 15 minutes

Ingredients:

- 1 avocado, peeled, pitted and chopped
- 1 large tomato, sliced
- ½ cup red onion, thinly sliced
- 8 romaine lettuce leaves, chopped
- 8 whole-wheat breads slices, toasted
- ¼ cup Dijon mustard

Directions:

1. In a large-sized bowl, blend together avocado, tomato, onion and lettuce.
2. Spread mustard over each slice evenly.
3. Place avocado mixture over 4 slices evenly.
4. Cover with remaining slices.
5. With a knife, carefully cut the sandwiches diagonally and serve.

Nutritional Information per Serving:

Calories: 242
Fat: 13g
Net Carbohydrates: 21.6g
Carbohydrates: 29.6g
Fiber: 8g
Sugar: 4g
Protein: 8.8g
Sodium: 268mg

Spinach & Tomato Sandwiches

Serves: 4 individuals
Preparation Time: 15 minutes
Cooking Time: 6 minutes

Ingredients:

- 4 multi-grain sandwich thins
- 4 teaspoons olive oil
- 1 tablespoon snipped fresh rosemary
- 4 eggs
- 2 cups fresh baby spinach
- 1 medium tomato, cut into 8 slices
- Salt and ground black pepper, as needed

Directions:

1. Preheat your oven to 375 °F.
2. Split each sandwich thin.
3. Brush cut sides of each sandwich thin with 2 teaspoons of olive oil.
4. Arrange the sandwich thins onto a large-sized baking sheet.
5. Bake for approximately 5 minutes.
6. Meanwhile, in a large-sized wok, heat the remaining 2 teaspoons of olive oil with rosemary over medium-high heat.
7. Break 1 egg into wok and cook for approximately 1 minute.
8. With a spatula, break the egg yolk.
9. Flip the egg and cook for approximately 1-2 minutes or until done.
10. Transfer the egg onto a plate.
11. Repeat with the remaining egg.
12. Place the bottom halves of sandwich thins onto serving plates.
13. Divide spinach among sandwich thins and top each with tomato slices, egg and 1 tablespoon of feta cheese.
14. Sprinkle each sandwich with salt and black pepper.
15. Top with the remaining sandwich thin halves and serve.

Nutritional Information per Serving

Calories: 217
Fat: 10.3g
Net Carbohydrates: 18g
Carbohydrates: 24.2g
Fiber: 6.2g
Sugar: 2.6g
Protein: 10.4g
Sodium: 320mg

Green Peas Sandwiches

Serves: 4 individuals
Preparation Time: 10 minutes

Ingredients:

- 1 cup boiled green peas, mashed slightly
- 1 tablespoon olive oil
- ½ cup low-fat feta cheese, crumbled
- 1 tablespoon fresh lemon juice
- 2 tablespoons fresh mint leaves, chopped
- 8 whole-wheat breads slices, toasted

Directions:

1. In a bowl, blend together peas, oil, feta, lemon juice, mint, salt and pepper.
2. Spread the peas mixture over 4 bread slices evenly.
3. Cover with remaining 4 bread slices.
4. Cut the sandwiches in half and serve.

Nutritional Information per Serving:

Calories: 204
Fat: 7.8g
Net Carbohydrates: 21.2g
Carbohydrates: 27g
Fiber: 5.8g
Sugar: 3.8g
Protein: 11.6g
Sodium: 288mg

Veggie Sandwiches

Serves: 4 individuals
Preparation Time: 15 minutes

Ingredients:

- 1 large cucumber, sliced
- ½ cup onion, thinly sliced
- 1 cup romaine lettuce leaves, chopped
- ½ cup fat-free plain yogurt
- ¼ tablespoon fresh lemon juice
- ¼ teaspoon ground cumin
- Salt and ground black pepper, as needed
- 8 whole-wheat breads slices, toasted

Directions:

1. In a large-sized bowl, blend together cucumber, onion, lettuce, yogurt, lemon juice and spices.
2. Spread mayonnaise over each slice evenly.
3. Divide the lettuce mixture over 4 slices evenly.
4. Cover with remaining slices.
5. Cut each sandwich in half and serve.

Nutritional Information per Serving:

Calories: 236
Fat: 10g
Net Carbohydrates: 27.8g
Carbohydrates: 30g
Fiber: 2.2g
Sugar: 3.4g
Protein: 5.2g
Sodium: 248mg

Chicken Sandwiches

Serves: 2 individuals
Preparation Time: 15 minutes
Cooking Time: 16 minutes

Ingredients:

- Olive oil cooking spray
- ½ cup onion, sliced

- 1 garlic clove, minced
- 4 whole-wheat breads slices
- ¼ cup low-fat cheddar cheese, shredded
- 2 lettuce leaves, torn
- ½ cup cooked chicken, shredded

Directions:
1. Grease a non-stick wok with cooking spray and heat it over medium-low heat.
2. Add in onion and garlic and cook for approximately 10 minutes, stirring occasionally.
3. Arrange 2 bread slices onto a smooth surface.
4. Sprinkle about 2 tablespoons of cheese over each slice evenly.
5. Arrange lettuce over each slice, followed by onion mixture and chicken.
6. Sprinkle with remaining cheese evenly.
7. Cover with remaining 2 bread slices.
8. Again, grease the same non-stick wok with cooking spray and heat over medium heat.
9. Add the sandwiches and cook for approximately 3 minutes per side.
10. Cut each sandwich in half and serve.

Nutritional Information per Serving:

Calories: 172
Fat: 6.4g
Net Carbohydrates: 11.4g
Carbohydrates: 12.6g
Fiber: 1.2g
Sugar: 2.2g
Protein: 15.4g
Sodium: 208mg

Turkey Sandwiches
Serves: 4 individuals
Preparation Time: 10 minutes
Cooking Time: 6 minutes

Ingredients:
- 8 whole-wheat breads slices
- 1 cup low-fat feta cheese, shredded
- 2 cups fresh spinach leaves, torn
- 8 (¼-inch thick) tomato slices
- 1 cup cooked turkey, shredded

Directions:
1. Arrange 4 bread slices onto a smooth surface.
2. Sprinkle about 2 tablespoons of cheese over each slice evenly.
3. Arrange ½ cup of spinach over each slice followed by 2 tomatoes slices, 2 tablespoons of onion mixture and 2 tablespoons of turkey meat.
4. Sprinkle with remaining cheese evenly.
5. Cover with remaining 4 bread slices.
6. Heat the greased non-stick wok over medium heat and cook the sandwiches for approximately 3 minutes per side.

7. With a knife, carefully cut the sandwiches diagonally and serve.

Nutritional Information per Serving:

Calories: 302
Fat: 9.8g
Net Carbohydrates: 23.4g
Carbohydrates: 28.4g
Fiber: 5g
Sugar: 4.8g
Protein: 26.4g
Sodium: 244mg

Tuna Sandwiches
Serves: 2 individuals
Preparation Time: 10 minutes

Ingredients:
- 1 (5-ounce) can water-packed tuna, drained
- 1 medium apple, peeled, cored and chopped
- 3 tablespoons plain Greek yogurt
- 1 teaspoon mustard
- ½ teaspoon organic honey
- 4 whole-wheat bread slices
- 2 lettuce leaves

Directions:
1. In a bowl, add the tuna, apple, yogurt, mustard and honey and stir to blend well.
2. Spread about ½ cup of the tuna mix over each of 3 bread slices.
3. Top each sandwich with 1 lettuce leaf.
4. Close with the remaining 3 bread slices.
5. Cut the sandwiches in half and serve.

Nutritional Information per Serving

Calories: 283
Fat: 4g
Net Carbohydrates: 34g
Carbohydrates: 40.2g
Fiber: 6.2g
Sugar: 16.4g
Protein: 26.6g
Sodium: 295mg

Crab Sandwiches
Serves: 4 individuals
Preparation Time: 15 minutes
Cooking Time: 6 minutes

Ingredients:
- 8 ounces crabmeat
- ¼ cup bell pepper, seeded and chopped
- 1/3 cup celery, finely chopped
- 1 scallion, finely chopped
- 1 tablespoon low-fat mayonnaise
- 4 teaspoons fresh lemon juice

- Ground black pepper, as needed
- 4 whole-wheat English muffins, halved and toasted
- ½ cup low-fat Parmesan cheese, shredded

Directions:
1. Preheat the broiler of oven to high.
2. In a large-sized bowl, blend together all ingredients except for muffins and cheese.
3. Arrange the English muffins onto a baking tray.
4. Place about ¼ cup of crabmeat mixture over each muffin half and sprinkle with cheese.
5. Broil for approximately 3-5 minutes per side.
6. Serve warm.

Nutritional Information per Serving:
Calories: 237
Fat: 5g
Net Carbohydrates: 32.6g
Carbohydrates: 37.7g
Fiber: 5.1g
Sugar: 9.8g
Protein: 13g
Sodium: 145mg

CHAPTER 9:
Snacks & Appetizer Recipes

Berries Gazpacho

Serves: 6 individuals
Preparation Time: 15 minutes

Ingredients:
- 2 cups fat-free plain yogurt
- ½ cup fresh orange juice
- 2 pounds mixed fresh berries
- ¼-1/3 cup organic honey
- 1 teaspoon organic vanilla extract

Directions:
1. Add all the ingredients in a high-powered blender and pulse until smooth.
2. Transfer the soup into a large-sized bowl.
3. Cover the bowl and refrigerate to chill for at least 2-3 hours before serving.

Nutritional Information per Serving:
Calories: 177
Fat: 0.7g
Net Carbohydrates: 32.4g
Carbohydrates: 37.9g
Fiber: 5.5g
Sugar: 24.2g
Protein: 4.6g
Sodium: 58mg

Apple & Almond Gazpacho

Serves: 6 individuals
Preparation Time: 15 minutes

Ingredients:
- 1 cup blanched almonds, soaked overnight in water and drained
- 2 stale whole-wheat bread slices, cut into cubes
- 1 apple, peeled, cored and chopped
- 1 small garlic clove
- 1 cup cold water
- 1-2 teaspoons apple cider vinegar
- Salt, as needed
- ¼ cup olive oil

Directions:
1. Place the stale bread in a high-powered blender, add almonds, bread cubes, apple, garlic, water, vinegar and salt and pulse until smooth.
2. While the motor is running, slowly add in the olive oil and pulse until smooth.
3. Transfer the almond soup mixture into a serving bowl and place in the refrigerator to chill before serving.

Nutritional Information per Serving:
Calories: 203
Fat: 16.8g
Net Carbohydrates: 8.8g
Carbohydrates: 12.2g

Fiber: 3.4g
Sugar: 4.8g
Protein: 4.6g
Sodium: 68mg

Strawberry & Veggie Gazpacho

Serves: 4 individuals
Preparation Time: 15 minutes

Ingredients:
- 1½ pounds fresh strawberries, hulled and sliced, plus extra for garnishing
- ½ cup red bell pepper, seeded and chopped
- 1 small cucumber, peeled, seeded, and chopped
- ¼ cup onion, chopped
- ¼ cup fresh basil leaves
- 1 small garlic clove, chopped
- ¼ small jalapeño pepper, seeded and chopped
- 1 tablespoon olive oil
- 2 tablespoons apple cider vinegar

Directions:
1. In a high-speed blender, add 1½ pounds of the strawberries and remaining ingredients and pulse until blended thoroughly and smooth.
2. Transfer the gazpacho into a large-sized serving bowl.
3. Cover the bowl of gazpacho and refrigerate for approximately 4 hours before serving.

Nutritional Information per Serving:
Calories: 106
Fat: 4.2g
Net Carbohydrates: 13.6g
Carbohydrates: 17.8g
Fiber: 4.2g
Sugar: 0.7g
Protein: 1.9g
Sodium: 4mg

Stuffed Okra Fries

Serves: 6 individuals
Preparation Time: 15 minutes
Cooking Time: 35 minutes

Ingredients:
- 2 tablespoons olive oil, divided
- 3 tablespoons creole seasoning
- ½ teaspoon ground turmeric
- 1 teaspoon water
- 1 pound okra, trimmed and slit in middle

Directions:
1. Preheat your oven to 450 °F.
2. Line a baking sheet with a piece of foil and then grease it with 1 tablespoon of oil.

3. In a large-sized bowl, blend together creole seasoning, turmeric and water.
4. Fill the slits of okra with turmeric mixture.
5. Place the okra onto prepared baking sheet and spread in a single layer.
6. Bake for approximately 30-35 minutes, flipping once halfway through.
7. Serve immediately.

Nutritional Information per Serving:
Calories: 71
Fat: 4.8g
Net Carbohydrates: 3.3g
Carbohydrates: 5.8g
Fiber: 2.5g
Sugar: 1.1g
Protein: 1.5g
Sodium: 65mg

Parsnip Fries
Serves: 6 individuals
Preparation Time: 15 minutes
Cooking Time: 40 minutes

Ingredients:
- 2 tablespoons extra-virgin olive oil
- 1¼ pound small parsnips, peeled and quartered
- 1½ tablespoons fresh ginger, minced
- Salt and ground black pepper, as needed

Directions:
1. Preheat your oven to 325 °F.
2. In a 13x9-inch baking dish, spread the oil evenly.
3. Place the remaining ingredients over oil and toss to combine.
4. With a piece of foil, cover the baking dish and bake for approximately 40 minutes.
5. Serve immediately.

Nutritional Information per Serving:
Calories: 116
Fat: 5g
Net Carbohydrates: 13.2g
Carbohydrates: 18g
Fiber: 4.8g
Sugar: 4.6g
Protein: 1.3g
Sodium: 37mg

Sweet Potato Fries
Serves: 2 individuals
Preparation Time: 10 minutes
Cooking Time: 25 minutes

Ingredients:
- 1 large sweet potato, peeled and cut into wedges

- 1 teaspoon ground turmeric
- 1 teaspoon ground cinnamon
- Salt and ground black pepper, as needed
- 2 tablespoons extra-virgin olive oil

Directions:
1. Preheat your oven to 425 °F.
2. Line a baking sheet with a piece of foil.
3. In a large-sized bowl, add all ingredients and toss to combine.
4. Transfer the mixture into the prepared baking sheet and spread in an even layer.
5. Bake for approximately 25 minutes, flipping once after 15 minutes.
6. Serve immediately.

Nutritional Information per Serving
Calories: 199
Fat: 14.3g
Net Carbohydrates: 14.7g
Carbohydrates: 18.2g
Fiber: 3.5g
Sugar: 5.3g
Protein: 1.8g
Sodium: 146mg

Jicama Fries

Serves: 3 individuals
Preparation Time: 15 minutes
Cooking Time: 51 minutes

Ingredients:
- 1 medium jicama, peeled and cut into fries
- 3 tablespoons water
- ½ teaspoon ground turmeric
- ½ teaspoon ground cumin
- ½ teaspoon garlic powder
- ¼ teaspoon onion powder
- ¼ teaspoon smoked paprika
- Pinch of cayenne powder
- Salt and ground black pepper, as needed

Directions:
1. Preheat your oven to 400 °F.
2. Line a baking sheet with a piece of foil.
3. In a large-sized microwave-safe bowl, add jicama fries and water.
4. Cover the bowl and microwave for approximately 6 minutes.
5. Drain the water completely.
6. Add the spices and oil and toss to combine.
7. Transfer the mixture onto the prepared baking sheet and spread in an even layer.
8. Bake for approximately 35-45 minutes, flipping once halfway through.
9. Serve immediately.

Nutritional Information per Serving:
Calories: 89
Fat: 0.4g
Net Carbohydrates: 9.4g
Carbohydrates: 20.4g
Fiber: 11g
Sugar: 4.2g
Protein: 1.8g
Sodium: 61mg

Potato Sticks

Serves: 2 individuals
Preparation Time: 10 minutes
Cooking Time: 10 minutes

Ingredients:
- 1 large russet potato, peeled and cut into 1/8 inch thick sticks lengthwise
- 10 curry leaves
- ¼ teaspoon ground turmeric
- ¼ teaspoon red chili powder
- Salt, as needed
- 1 tablespoon olive oil

Directions:
1. Preheat your oven to 400 °F.
2. Line 2 baking sheets with parchment papers.

3. In a large-sized bowl, add all ingredients and toss to combine.
4. Divide the mixture onto prepared baking sheets and then spread in a single layer.
5. Bake for approximately 10 minutes.
6. Serve immediately.

Nutritional Information per Serving:
Calories: 204
Fat: 7.3g
Net Carbohydrates: 28.2g
Carbohydrates: 32.6g
Fiber: 4.2g
Sugar: 1.5g
Protein: 3.8g
Sodium: 92mg

Apple Chips

Serves: 8 individuals
Preparation Time: 15 minutes
Cooking Time: 2 hours

Ingredients:
- 2 tablespoons ground cinnamon
- 1 tablespoon ground ginger
- 1½ teaspoons ground cloves
- 1½ teaspoons ground nutmeg
- Salt and ground black pepper, as needed
- 3 Fuji apples, sliced thinly in rounds

Directions:
1. Preheat your oven to 200 °F.
2. Line a large-sized baking sheet with parchment paper.
3. In a bowl, blend together all spices, salt and black pepper.
4. Arrange the apple slices onto prepared baking sheet in a single layer.
5. Sprinkle the apple slices with spice mixture generously.
6. Bake for approximately 1 hour.
7. Flip the side of apple slices and sprinkle with spice mixture.
8. Bake for approximately 1 hour.
9. Remove the apple chips from oven and set aside to cool completely before serving.

Nutritional Information per Serving:
Calories: 71
Fat: 0.6g
Net Carbohydrates: 14.2g
Carbohydrates: 18.5g
Fiber: 4.3g
Sugar: 11.9g
Protein: 0.5g
Sodium: 3mg

Plantain Chips

Serves: 3 individuals
Preparation Time: 10 minutes
Cooking Time: 20 minutes

Ingredients:
- Olive oil cooking spray
- 2 plantains, peeled and sliced
- 1 teaspoon ground turmeric
- Salt, as needed
- 2 teaspoons coconut oil, melted

Directions:
1. Grease a microwave-safe dish with cooking spray.
2. In a large-sized bowl, add all ingredients and toss to combine.
3. Transfer the half of the mixture into the prepared dish.
4. Microwave on high for approximately 3 minutes.
5. Now, reduce the power to 50% and microwave for approximately 2 minutes.
6. Repeat with the remaining plantain mixture.

Nutritional Information per Serving:
Calories: 174
Fat: 14.2g
Net Carbohydrates: 35.6g
Carbohydrates: 38.5g
Fiber: 2.9g
Sugar: 17.9g
Protein: 1.6g
Sodium: 155mg

Spinach Chips

Serves: 2 individuals
Preparation Time: 10 minutes
Cooking Time: 8 minutes

Ingredients:
- 4 cups fresh spinach leaves
- 1-2 teaspoons extra-virgin olive oil
- Salt, as needed
- ½ teaspoon Italian seasoning

Directions:
1. Preheat your oven to 325 °F.
2. Line a large-sized baking sheet with parchment paper.
3. In a large-sized bowl, add spinach leaves and drizzle with oil.
4. With your hands, rub the spinach leaves until all the leaves are coated with oil.
5. Transfer the leaves onto the prepared baking sheet and spread in a single layer.
6. Sprinkle the spinach leaves with salt and Italian seasoning.
7. Bake for approximately 8 minutes.
8. Remove the baking sheet of chips from oven and set aside for approximately 5 minutes before serving.

Nutritional Information per Serving:
Calories: 37
Fat: 2.9g
Net Carbohydrates: 1g
Carbohydrates: 2.3g
Fiber: 1.3g
Sugar: 0.4g
Protein: 1.7g
Sodium: 125mg

Beet Greens Chips

Serves: 2 individuals
Preparation Time: 10 minutes
Cooking Time: 25 minutes

Ingredients:
- 4 cups beet greens, tough ribs removed
- Salt and ground black pepper, as needed
- 1 tablespoon olive oil

Directions:
1. Preheat your oven to 350 °F.
2. Line a large-sized baking sheet with parchment paper.
3. In a large-sized bowl, add all ingredients and toss to combine.
4. Transfer the leaves onto the prepared baking sheet and spread in a single layer.
5. Bake for approximately 25 minutes, flipping once after 15 minutes.
6. Remove the baking sheet of chips from oven and set aside for approximately 5 minutes before serving.

Nutritional Information per Serving:
Calories: 77
Fat: 7.1g
Net Carbohydrates: 0.5g
Carbohydrates: 3.3g
Fiber: 2.8g
Sugar: 0.4g
Protein: 1.7g
Sodium: 249mg

Beet Crackers

Serves: 15 individuals
Preparation Time: 20 minutes
Cooking Time: 50 minutes

Ingredients:
- Olive oil cooking spray
- 1 cup raw beets, chopped
- 3 tablespoons arrowroot flour
- 3 tablespoons coconut flour
- 2 egg whites
- 1 tablespoon coconut oil
- ¼ teaspoon ground turmeric
- 1/8 teaspoon cayenne powder
- Salt and ground black pepper, as needed

Directions:
1. Preheat your oven to 350 °F.
2. Grease a large-sized baking sheet with cooking spray.
3. In a clean food processor, add beets and pulse until just a puree form.
4. Add remaining ingredients and pulse until blended thoroughly.
5. Place a parchment paper onto a smooth surface.
6. Place the dough onto parchment paper and top with another paper.
7. With a rolling pin, roll the dough to 1/8-inch thickness.
8. Remove the parchment papers.
9. Place the rolled dough onto the prepared baking sheet.
10. Bake for approximately 40-50 minutes.
11. Remove the baking sheet of crackers from oven and place onto a wire rack to cool completely before serving.

Nutritional Information per Serving:
Calories: 28
Fat: 1.3g
Net Carbohydrates: 1.7g
Carbohydrates: 3g
Fiber: 1.3g
Sugar: 1.1g
Protein: 1.1g
Sodium: 31mg

Fruit Crackers

Serves: 15 individuals
Preparation Time: 20 minutes
Cooking Time: 12 hours

Ingredients:
- 8 carrots
- 1 orange, peeled
- 1 apple
- 1 (1-inch) piece fresh ginger
- 1 onion
- 1 cup chia seeds
- ½ cup sesame seeds
- 1 tablespoon ground turmeric
- Salt and ground black pepper, as needed

Directions:
1. In a juicer, add carrots and extract juice according to manufacturer's directions.
2. In a bowl, transfer the carrot juice and pulp.
3. Now, in juicer, add orange, apple and ginger and extract the juice.
4. Transfer the juice in the bowl with carrot juice and pulp.
5. In a clean food processor, add juice mixture and remaining ingredients and pulse until a puree forms.
6. Spread the mixture into 3 dehydrator trays evenly.
7. With a knife, score the size of crackers.
8. Set dehydrator at 115 °F.
9. Dehydrate for approximately 12 hours.
10. Remove the trays of crackers from dehydrator and place onto a wire rack to cool completely before serving.

Nutritional Information per Serving:
Calories: 90
Fat: 5.1g
Net Carbohydrates: 7.1g
Carbohydrates: 12g
Fiber: 4.9g
Sugar: 4.6g
Protein: 3g
Sodium: 35mg

Apple Leather

Serves: 4 individuals
Preparation Time: 15 minutes
Cooking Time: 12 hours 25 minutes

Ingredients:
- 1 cup water
- 8 cups apples, peeled, cored and chopped
- 1 tablespoon ground cinnamon
- 2 tablespoons fresh lemon juice

Directions:
1. In a large-sized saucepan, add water and apples over medium-low heat.
2. Simmer for approximately 10-15 minutes, stirring occasionally.
3. Remove the pan of apples from heat and set aside to cool slightly.
4. In a clean blender, add apple mixture and pulse until smooth.
5. Return the mixture into pan over medium-low heat.

6. Stir in cinnamon and lemon juice and simmer for approximately 10 minutes.
7. Transfer the mixture onto dehydrator trays and with the back of spoon smooth the top.
8. Set the dehydrator at 135 °F.
9. Dehydrate for approximately 10-12 hours.
10. Cut the apple leather into equal-sized rectangles.
11. Now, roll each rectangle to make fruit rolls and serve.

Nutritional Information per Serving:
Calories: 238
Fat: 0.9g
Net Carbohydrates: 51.4g
Carbohydrates: 63.1g
Fiber: 11.7g
Sugar: 46.6g
Protein: 1.3g
Sodium: 7mg

Spicy Popcorn

Serves: 2 individuals
Preparation Time: 10 minutes
Cooking Time: 2 minutes

Ingredients:
- 2 tablespoons coconut oil
- ½ cup popping corn
- 1 tablespoon olive oil
- 1 teaspoon ground turmeric
- ¼ teaspoon ground cumin
- ¼ teaspoon garlic powder
- Salt, as needed

Directions:
1. In a saucepan, melt coconut oil over medium-high heat.
2. Add popping corn and immediately cover the pan tightly.
3. Cook for approximately 1-2 minutes or until corn kernels start to pop, shaking the pan occasionally.
4. Remove the pan of popcorn from heat and transfer into a large-sized heatproof bowl.
5. Add in olive oil, spices and salt and mix well.
6. Serve immediately.

Nutritional Information per Serving:
Calories: 273
Fat: 21.8g
Net Carbohydrates: 14.8g
Carbohydrates: 19.1g
Fiber: 4.3g
Sugar: 0.1g
Protein: 2.7g
Sodium: 78mg

Spiced Almonds

Serves: 8 individuals
Preparation Time: 10 minutes
Cooking Time: 10 minutes

Ingredients:
- 2 cups whole almonds
- 1 tablespoon red chili powder
- ½ teaspoon ground cinnamon
- ½ teaspoon ground cumin
- ½ teaspoon ground coriander
- Salt and ground black pepper, as needed
- 1 tablespoon extra-virgin olive oil

Directions:
1. Preheat your oven to 350 °F.
2. Line a baking dish with parchment paper.
3. In a bowl, add all ingredients and toss to combine.
4. Transfer the almond mixture into prepared baking dish and spread in a single layer.
5. Roast for approximately 10 minutes, flipping once halfway through.
6. Remove the baking dish of almonds from oven and set aside to cool completely before serving.

Nutritional Information per Serving:
Calories: 156
Fat: 13.8g
Net Carbohydrates: 2.4g
Carbohydrates: 5.8g
Fiber: 3.4g
Sugar: 1.1g
Protein: 5.2g
Sodium: 29mg

Sweet & Spicy Cashews

Serves: 8 individuals
Preparation Time: 10 minutes
Cooking Time: 20 minutes

Ingredients:
- 2 cups cashews
- 2 teaspoons organic honey
- 1½ teaspoons smoked paprika
- ½ teaspoon chili flakes
- Salt, as needed
- 1 tablespoon fresh lemon juice
- 1 teaspoon olive oil

Directions:
1. Preheat your oven to 350 °F.
2. Line a large-sized baking dish with parchment paper.
3. In a large-sized bowl, add all ingredients and toss to combine.

4. Transfer the cashew mixture into prepared baking dish and spread in a single layer.
5. Roast for approximately 20 minutes, flipping once halfway through.
6. Remove the baking dish of cashews from oven and set aside to cool completely before serving.

Nutritional Information per Serving:
Calories: 212
Fat: 16.7g
Net Carbohydrates: 11.9g
Carbohydrates: 13.5g
Fiber: 1.6g
Sugar: 3.4g
Protein: 5.5g
Sodium: 26mg

Stuffed Cherry Tomatoes

Serves: 6 individuals
Preparation Time: 20 minutes

Ingredients:
- 2¼ cups cherry tomatoes
- 1 small avocado, peeled, pitted and chopped
- 2 tablespoons cashews, chopped
- 2 garlic cloves, chopped
- 1 jalapeño pepper, seeded and chopped
- 2 tablespoons fresh basil leaves
- 1 tablespoon fresh lemon juice

Directions:
1. With a small-sized sharp knife, cut the top of each tomato.
2. With a little scooper, remove the seeds from tomatoes, to create cups.
3. Arrange the tomatoes in large serving plates, cut side up.
4. In a clean food processor, add remaining all ingredients and pulse until smooth.
5. Carefully fill each tomato cup with avocado mixture.

6. Serve immediately.

Nutritional Information per Serving:
Calories: 70
Fat: 5.2g
Net Carbohydrates: 3.4g
Carbohydrates: 5.7g
Fiber: 2.3g
Sugar: 2.2g
Protein: 1.5g
Sodium: 6mg

Green Deviled Eggs

Serves: 6 individuals
Preparation Time: 10 minutes

Ingredients:
- 6 hard-boiled large organic eggs
- 1 medium avocado, peeled, pitted and chopped
- 2 teaspoons fresh lime juice
- Salt, as needed

Directions:
1. Peel the eggs and with a knife, slice them in half vertically.
2. Carefully scoop out the yolks from each egg half.
3. In a bowl, add half of egg yolks, avocado, lime juice and salt and with a fork, mash until blended thoroughly.
4. Scoop the avocado mixture in the egg halves evenly and serve.

Nutritional Information per Serving:
Calories: 120
Fat: 9.6g
Net Carbohydrates: 0.8g
Carbohydrates: 2.4g
Fiber: 1.6g
Sugar: 0.5g
Protein: 6.7g
Sodium: 99mg

CHAPTER 10:
Dessert Recipes

Pineapple Sticks

Serves: 8 individuals
Preparation Time: 10 minutes
Ingredients:
- ¼ cup fresh orange juice
- ¾ cup unsweetened coconut, shredded and toasted
- 8 (3x1-inch) fresh pineapple pieces

Directions:
1. Line a baking sheet with wax paper.
2. In a shallow dish, place the pineapple juice.
3. In another shallow dish, place the coconut.
4. Insert 1 wooden skewer in each pineapple piece from the narrow end.
5. Dip each pineapple piece in juice and then coat with coconut evenly.
6. Arrange the pineapple sticks onto prepared baking sheet in a single layer.
7. Cover and refrigerate for approximately 1-2 hours before serving.

Nutritional Information per Serving:
Calories: 58
Fat: 2.6g
Net Carbohydrates: 7.9g
Carbohydrates: 9.4g
Fiber: 1.5g
Sugar: 6.7g
Protein: 0.6g
Sodium: 2mg

Cinnamon Peaches

Serves: 2 individuals
Preparation Time: 10 minutes
Cooking Time: 10 minutes
Ingredients:
- Olive oil cooking spray
- 2 medium peaches, halved and pitted
- 1/8 teaspoon ground cinnamon

Directions:
1. Preheat the grill to medium-low heat.
2. Grease the grill grate with cooking spray.
3. Arrange the peach slices onto the grill, cut-side down.
4. Grill for approximately 3-5 minutes per side or until desired doneness.
5. Sprinkle with cinnamon and serve.

Nutritional Information per Serving
Calories: 60
Fat: 0.4g
Net Carbohydrates: 11.8g
Carbohydrates: 14.2g
Fiber: 2.4g
Sugar: 13.9g
Protein: 1.4g
Sodium: 0mg

Spiced Apples

Serves: 4 individuals
Preparation Time: 10 minutes
Cooking Time: 18 minutes

Ingredients:
- 4 tart apples, cored
- ¼ cup coconut oil, softened
- 4 teaspoons ground cinnamon
- 1/8 teaspoon ground ginger
- 1/8 teaspoon ground nutmeg

Directions:
1. Preheat your oven to 350 °F.
2. Fill each apple with 1 tablespoon of coconut oil and sprinkle with spices evenly.
3. Arrange the apples onto a baking sheet.
4. Bake for approximately 12-18 minutes.
5. Serve warm.

Nutritional Information per Serving:
Calories: 237
Fat: 14.1g
Net Carbohydrates: 25.8g
Carbohydrates: 31.8g
Fiber: 6g
Sugar: 23.2g
Protein: 0.7g
Sodium: 2mg

Frozen Mango Feast

Serves: 4 individuals
Preparation Time: 10 minutes

Ingredients:
- 3 cups frozen mango, peeled, pitted, and chopped
- 1 tablespoon fresh mint leaves
- 2 tablespoons fresh lime juice
- ½ cup chilled water

Directions:
1. In a high-powered blender, add all ingredients and pulse until smooth.
2. Transfer into serving bowls and serve immediately.

Nutritional Information per Serving:
Calories: 76
Fat: 0.5g
Net Carbohydrates: 17.2g
Carbohydrates: 19.4g
Fiber: 2.2g
Sugar: 16.9g
Protein: 1.1g
Sodium: 4mg

Strawberry & Citrus Granita

Serves: 5 individuals
Preparation Time: 15 minutes

Ingredients:
- 12 ounces fresh strawberries, hulled
- 1 grapefruit, peeled, seeded and sectioned

- 2 oranges, peeled, seeded and sectioned
- ¼ of a lemon
- ¼ cup organic honey

Directions:
1. In a juicer, add strawberries, grapefruit, oranges and lemon and process according to manufacturer's directions.
2. In a small-sized heavy-bottomed saucepan, add 1½ cups of the fruit juice and honey over medium heat and cook for approximately 5 minutes, stirring continuously.
3. Remove the pan of juice mixture from heat and stir in the remaining juice.
4. Set aside to cool for approximately 30 minutes.
5. Transfer the juice mixture into an 8x8-inch glass baking dish.
6. Freeze for approximately 4 hours, scraping after every 30 minutes.

Nutritional Information per Serving:
Calories: 116
Fat: 0.3g
Net Carbohydrates: 26.5g
Carbohydrates: 30g
Fiber: 3.5g
Sugar: 25.9g
Protein: 1.4g
Sodium: 1mg

Spinach Sorbet
Serves: 4 individuals
Preparation Time: 15 minutes

Ingredients:
- 3 cups fresh spinach, torn
- 1 tablespoon fresh basil leaves
- ½ of avocado, peeled, pitted and chopped
- ¾ cup unsweetened almond milk
- 20 drops liquid stevia
- 1 teaspoon almonds, chopped very finely
- 1 teaspoon organic vanilla extract
- 1 cup ice cubes

Directions:
1. In a clean blender, add spinach and remaining ingredients and pulse until creamy and smooth.
2. Transfer into an ice cream maker and process according to manufacturer's directions.
3. Transfer into an airtight container and freeze for at least 4-5 hours before serving.

Nutritional Information per Serving:
Calories: 375
Fat: 16g
Net Carbohydrates: 2.5g
Carbohydrates: 5.7g
Fiber: 3.2g

Sugar: 1.9g
Protein: 2.3g
Sodium: 26mg

Pumpkin & Dates Ice Cream
Serves: 8 individuals
Preparation Time: 10 minutes

Ingredients:
- 1 (15-ounce) can sugar-free pumpkin puree
- ½ cup dates, pitted and chopped
- 2 (14-ounce) cans unsweetened coconut milk
- ½ teaspoon organic vanilla extract
- 1½ teaspoons pumpkin pie spice
- ½ teaspoon ground cinnamon
- Pinch of salt

Directions:
1. In a high-powered blender, add pumpkin puree and remaining ingredients and pulse until smooth.
2. Transfer into an airtight container and freeze for approximately 1-2 hours.
3. Now, transfer into an ice-cream maker and process according to manufacturer's directions.
4. Return the ice-cream into airtight container and freeze for approximately 1-2 hours.

Nutritional Information per Serving:
Calories: 200
Fat: 13.9g
Net Carbohydrates: 12.9g
Carbohydrates: 15.5g
Fiber: 2.6g
Sugar: 11.3g
Protein: 2.1g
Sodium: 53mg

Banana & Avocado Mousse
Serves: 4 individuals
Preparation Time: 15 minutes
Ingredients:
- 2 cups bananas, peeled and chopped
- 2 ripe avocados, peeled, pitted and chopped
- 1 teaspoon fresh lime zest, grated finely
- 1 teaspoon fresh lemon zest, grated finely
- ½ cup fresh lime juice
- ½ cup fresh lemon juice
- 1/3 cup organic honey

Directions:
1. In a clean blender, add bananas and remaining ingredients and pulse until smooth.
2. Transfer the mousse in 4 serving glasses and refrigerate to chill for approximately 3-4 hours.

Nutritional Information per Serving:
Calories: 308

Fat: 14.3g
Net Carbohydrates: 40.6g
Carbohydrates: 47.6g
Fiber: 7g
Sugar: 33.4g
Protein: 2.5g
Sodium: 12mg

Chocolaty Avocado Mousse

Serves: 6 individuals
Preparation Time: 10 minutes
Ingredients:
- 2 ripe avocados, peeled, pitted and chopped
- ½ cup unsweetened coconut milk
- ½ cup cacao powder
- 1 teaspoon ground cinnamon
- ¼ teaspoon ground ancho chili
- 1/3 cup organic honey
- 2 teaspoons vanilla extract

Directions:
1. In a clean blender, add avocados and remaining ingredients and pulse until smooth.
2. Transfer the mousse in 4 serving glasses and refrigerate to chill for approximately 3 hours.

Nutritional Information per Serving:
Calories: 221
Fat: 15.3g
Net Carbohydrates: 18.1g
Carbohydrates: 24.5g
Fiber: 5.9g
Sugar: 16.6g
Protein: 2.8g
Sodium: 7mg

Chocolaty Chia Pudding

Serves: 6 individuals
Preparation Time: 15 minutes
Ingredients:
- 7-9 dates, pitted and chopped
- 1½ cups unsweetened almond milk
- 1/3 cup chia seeds
- ¼ cup cacao powder
- ½ teaspoon ground cinnamon
- 1/8 teaspoon salt
- ½ teaspoon organic vanilla extract

Directions:
1. In a clean blender, add dates and remaining ingredients and pulse until smooth.
2. Transfer the pudding in 6 serving glasses and refrigerate to chill completely before serving.

Nutritional Information per Serving:
Calories: 73
Fat: 3.8g
Net Carbohydrates: 8g
Carbohydrates: 12.3g
Fiber: 4.3g

Sugar: 6.2g
Protein: 2.5g
Sodium: 96mg

Pumpkin Custard

Serves: 6 individuals
Preparation Time: 15 minutes
Cooking Time: 1 hour

Ingredients:
- 1 cup canned pumpkin
- 1 teaspoon ground cinnamon
- ¼ teaspoon ground ginger
- 1/8 teaspoon ground cloves
- 2 pinches of nutmeg, grated freshly
- Pinch of salt
- 2 organic eggs
- 1 cup unsweetened coconut milk
- 8-10 drops liquid stevia
- 1 teaspoon organic vanilla extract

Directions:
1. Preheat your oven to 350 °F.
2. In a large-sized bowl, blend together the pumpkin, spices and salt.
3. In another large-sized bowl, add the eggs and whisk well.
4. Add coconut milk, stevia and vanilla extract and whisk until blended thoroughly.
5. Add egg mixture into the bowl of pumpkin mixture and mix until blended thoroughly.
6. Transfer the mixture into 6 ramekins.
7. Arrange the ramekins into a baking dish,
8. Add enough water in the baking dish about 2-inch high around the ramekins.
9. Bake for approximately 1 hour.
10. Serve warm.

Nutritional Information per Serving:
Calories: 130
Fat: 11.1g
Net Carbohydrates: 43.9g
Carbohydrates: 50g
Fiber: 6.1g
Sugar: 2.3g
Protein: 3.3g
Sodium: 56mg

Chocolate Custard

Serves: 6 individuals
Preparation Time: 15 minutes
Cooking Time: 35 minutes

Ingredients:
- Olive oil cooking spray
- 1½ (14-ounce) cans unsweetened coconut milk
- 5 large organic eggs
- ½ cup organic honey

- 1 tablespoon vanilla extract
- 3 tablespoons cocoa powder
- 2 tablespoons hot water
- Pinch of ground cinnamon
- Pinch of ground nutmeg

Directions:
1. Preheat your oven to 325 °F.
2. Grease a casserole dish with cooking spray
3. In a large-sized bowl, add coconut milk, eggs and honey and whisk until blended thoroughly.
4. In a small-sized bowl, add cocoa powder and hot water and mix until a paste forms.
5. Add chocolate paste in eggs mixture and stir to blend.
6. Transfer the mixture into prepared casserole dish evenly and sprinkle with cinnamon and nutmeg.
7. Arrange the casserole dish into a large-sized baking dish.
8. Pour the boiling water in baking dish about half way of the casserole dish.
9. Bake for approximately 35 minutes.
10. Serve warm.

Nutritional Information per Serving:
Calories: 307
Fat: 18.2g
Net Carbohydrates: 27g
Carbohydrates: 27.9g
Fiber: 0.9g
Sugar: 26.3g
Protein: 7.1g
Sodium: 91mg

Strawberry Soufflé
Serves: 6 individuals
Preparation Time: 15 minutes
Cooking Time: 12 minutes

Ingredients:
- 18 ounces fresh strawberries, hulled
- 1/3 cup organic honey, divided
- 5 organic egg whites, divided
- 4 teaspoons fresh lemon juice

Directions:
1. Preheat your oven to 350 °F.
2. In a clean blender, ad strawberries and pulse until a puree forms.
3. Through a strainer, strain the strawberry puree and discard the seeds.
4. In a large-sized bowl, add strawberry puree, 3 tablespoons of honey, 2 egg whites and lemon juice and pulse until frothy and light.
5. In another bowl, add remaining egg whites and whisk until frothy.

6. While beating gradually, add remaining honey and whisk until stiff peaks form.
7. Gently fold the egg whites into strawberry mixture.
8. Transfer the mixture into 6 large ramekins evenly.
9. Arrange the ramekins onto a baking sheet.
10. Bake for approximately 10-12 minutes.
11. Remove the ramekins from oven and serve immediately.

Nutritional Information per Serving:
Calories: 100
Fat: 0.3g
Net Carbohydrates: 20.5g
Carbohydrates: 22.3g
Fiber: 1.8g
Sugar: 19.8g
Protein: 3.7g
Sodium: 30mg

Apple & Cranberry Crisp
Serves: 6 individuals
Preparation Time: 15 minutes
Cooking Time: 48 minutes
Ingredients:
For Filling:

- 2 tablespoons coconut oil
- 2 tablespoons organic honey
- 2 teaspoons ground cinnamon
- ½ teaspoon ground nutmeg
- ¼ teaspoon ground ginger
- ¼ teaspoon ground cloves
- 1½ pound apples, peeled, cored and chopped
- ½ cup fresh cranberries

For Topping:

- 1 cup coconut, shredded
- ½ cup coconut palm sugar
- ¼ cup coconut oil, softened
- 3 tablespoons tapioca starch
- 2 tablespoons coconut flour
- ½ teaspoon ground cinnamon
- ¼ teaspoon ground nutmeg
- Pinch of salt

Directions:
1. Preheat your oven to 350 °F.
2. For filling: in a saucepan, blend together coconut oil, honey and spices.
3. Place the pan of oil mixture over low heat and cook for approximately 2-3 minutes, stirring continuously.
4. Remove the pan of oil mixture from heat and transfer the mixture into a bowl.
5. Add apples and cranberries and toss to combine.
6. Now place the mixture into an 8x8-inch pie dish.

7. For topping: in a medium-sized glass bowl, add all ingredients and mix until a crumbly mixture forms.
8. Place the topping mixture over filling evenly.
9. Bake for approximately 35-45 minutes or until top becomes golden brown.
10. Serve warm.

Nutritional Information per Serving:
Calories: 310
Fat: 18.5g
Net Carbohydrates: 34.6g
Carbohydrates: 39g
Fiber: 4.4g
Sugar: 24.9g
Protein: 1g
Sodium: 67mg

Tropical Fruit Crisp

Serves: 8 individuals
Preparation Time: 15 minutes
Cooking Time: 20 minutes

Ingredients:
For Filling:
- 2 tablespoons coconut oil
- 2 tablespoons coconut sugar
- 1 large mango, peeled, pitted and chopped
- 3-4 cups fresh pineapple, peeled and cut into chunks
- 1/8 teaspoon ground cinnamon
- 1/8 teaspoon ground ginger

For Topping:
- ¾ cup almonds
- 1/3 cup unsweetened coconut, shredded
- ½ teaspoon ground allspice
- ½ teaspoon ground cinnamon
- ½ teaspoon ground ginger

Directions:
1. Preheat your oven to 375 °F.
2. For filling: in a saucepan, melt coconut oil over medium-low heat and cook coconut sugar for approximately 1-2 minutes, stirring continuously.
3. Stir in remaining ingredients and cook for approximately 5 minutes.
4. Remove the pan of filling from heat and transfer the mixture into a baking dish.
5. Meanwhile, for topping in a clean food processor, add all ingredients and pulse until a coarse meal forms.
6. Place the topping over filling evenly.
7. Bake for approximately 13-15 minutes or until top becomes golden brown.
8. Remove the baking dish of crisp from oven and set aside to cool slightly.
9. Serve warm.

Nutritional Information per Serving:
Calories: 160
Fat: 9.2g
Net Carbohydrates: 17g
Carbohydrates: 20g
Fiber: 3g
Sugar: 15.4g
Protein: 2.7g
Sodium: 2mg

Cherry Cobbler

Serves: 4 individuals
Preparation Time: 10 minutes
Cooking Time: 25 minutes

Ingredients:
- 2 cups fresh cherries, pitted
- ¼ cup plus 1 tablespoon coconut palm sugar, divided
- ¼ cup pecans, chopped
- ¼ cup unsweetened coconut, shredded
- ¼ cup coconut flour
- 1 tablespoon arrowroot flour
- ½ teaspoon ground cinnamon
- Pinch of salt

Directions:
1. Preheat your oven to 375 °F.
2. In a 7x5-inch baking dish, place the cherries.
3. Place ¼ cup of coconut sugar over cherries evenly.
4. In a bowl, add 1 tablespoon of coconut sugar and remaining ingredients.
5. Spread pecan mixture over cherries evenly.
6. Bake for approximately 20-25 minutes.
7. Serve warm.

Nutritional Information per Serving:
Calories: 166
Fat: 7.2g
Net Carbohydrates: 22.6g
Carbohydrates: 25.8g
Fiber: 3.2g
Sugar: 19.2g
Protein: 2.2g
Sodium: 69mg

Pumpkin Pie

Serves: 8 individuals
Preparation Time: 15 minutes
Cooking Time: 1 hour 5 minutes

Ingredients:

For Crust:
- 2½ cups walnuts
- 1 teaspoon baking soda
- Salt, as needed
- 2 tablespoons coconut oil, melted

For Filling:
- 1 (15-ounce) can sugar-free pumpkin puree
- 1 tablespoon arrowroot powder
- ½ teaspoon ground nutmeg
- ½ teaspoon ground cinnamon
- ¼ teaspoon ground ginger
- ¼ teaspoon ground cardamom
- ¼ teaspoon ground cloves
- Pinch of salt
- 1 cup unsweetened coconut milk
- 3 eggs, beaten
- 3 tablespoons organic honey

Directions:
1. Preheat your oven to 350 °F.
2. For crust: in a clean food processor, add walnuts, baking soda and salt and pulse until finely ground.
3. Now add the coconut oil and pulse until well blended.
4. Place the crust mixture into a 9-inch pie dish.
5. With the back of a spatula, smooth the surface of crust.
6. Arrange the pie dish onto a baking sheet.
7. Bake for approximately 15 minutes.
8. Meanwhile, for filling in a large-sized bowl, add all ingredients and mix until well blended.
9. Remove the crust from oven.
10. Place the mixture over the crust.
11. Bake for approximately 50 minutes.
12. Remove the pie dish from oven and place onto the wire rack to cool for approximately 10 minutes.
13. Freeze for approximately 3-4 hours before serving.

Nutritional Information per Serving:
Calories: 387
Fat: 32.4g
Net Carbohydrates: 12.4g
Carbohydrates: 16.8g
Fiber: 4.4g
Sugar: 9.6g
Protein: 12.5g
Sodium: 215mg

No-Bake Cheesecake

Serves: 12 individuals
Preparation Time: 20 minutes

Ingredients:

For Crust:
- 1 cup dates, pitted and chopped
- 1 cup raw almonds
- 2-3 tablespoons unsweetened coconut, shredded

For Filling:
- 3½ cups cashews, soaked overnight
- ½ cup coconut oil, melted
- 2 tablespoons fresh lemon rind, grated finely
- ¾ cup fresh lemon juice
- ¾ cup organic honey
- 10 drops liquid stevia
- 1 teaspoon organic vanilla extract
- Salt, as needed
- 1 lemon, sliced thinly

Directions:
1. Place the dates, almonds and coconut in a clean food processor and pulse until mixture just starts to blend.
2. Transfer the mixture into a greased springform pan.
3. With the back of spatula, smooth the surface of crust.
4. In a clean food processor, add cashews and oil and pulse until blended thoroughly.
5. Add the remaining ingredients except lemon slices and pulse until creamy and smooth.
6. Place the mixture over crust evenly.
7. With the back of spatula, smooth the surface of filling.
8. Refrigerate for approximately 1 hour.
9. Remove from the refrigerator and garnish with lemon slices.
10. Cut into desired sized slices and serve.

Nutritional Information per Serving:
Calories: 468
Fat: 32g
Net Carbohydrates: 40.5g
Carbohydrates: 44.2g
Fiber: 3.7g
Sugar: 29.6g
Protein: 8.4g
Sodium: 11mg

Pineapple & Cherry Upside-Down Cake

Serves: 6 individuals
Preparation Time: 15 minutes
Cooking Time: 50 minutes

Ingredients:

- 5 tablespoons organic honey, divided
- 2 (½-inch thick) fresh pineapple slices
- 15 fresh sweet cherries
- 1 cup almond flour
- ½ teaspoon baking powder
- 2 organic eggs
- 3 tablespoons coconut oil, melted
- 1 teaspoon organic vanilla extract
- Fresh cherries, for garnishing

Directions:

1. Preheat your oven to 350 °F.
2. In an 8-inch round cake pan, place about 1½ tablespoons of honey evenly.
3. Arrange the pineapple slices and 15 cherries over honey in your desired pattern.
4. Bake for approximately 15 minutes.
5. In a bowl, blend together almond flour and baking powder.
6. In another bowl, add eggs and remaining honey and whisk until creamy.
7. In the bowl of egg mixture, add coconut oil and vanilla extract and whisk until well blended.
8. Add flour mixture into egg mixture and mix until well blended.
9. Remove the cake pan from oven.
10. Place the flour mixture over pineapple and cherries evenly.
11. Bake for approximately 35 minutes.
12. Remove the pan of cake from oven and set aside to cool for approximately 10 minutes.
13. Carefully remove the cake from pan and place onto a serving plate.
14. Cut into desired-sized slices and serve.

Nutritional Information per Serving

Calories: 180
Fat: 10.6g
Net Carbohydrates: 19.2g
Carbohydrates: 20.4g
Fiber: 1.2g
Sugar: 18.6g
Protein: 3.3g
Sodium: 23mg

Chocolaty Pumpkin Cake

Serves: 8 individuals
Preparation Time: 20 minutes
Cooking Time: 40 minutes

Ingredients:

- Olive oil cooking spray

For Cake:

- 1 cup unsweetened dark chocolate chips
- 1/3 cup coconut oil, softened
- 1/3 cup coconut flour
- 2 tablespoons unsweetened almond milk
- ¼ cup organic honey
- ¾ cup sugar-free pumpkin puree
- 3 organic eggs
- ½ teaspoon ground nutmeg
- ½ teaspoon ground cinnamon
- ¼ teaspoon ground ginger

For Frosting:

- ½ (14-ounce) can unsweetened coconut milk
- 2 tablespoon pumpkin puree
- 1 teaspoon organic honey
- Pinch of ground cinnamon

Directions:

1. Preheat your oven to 350 °F.
2. Grease an 8x8-inch glass baking dish with cooking spray
3. In a microwave-safe bowl, add chocolate chips and microwave on low for approximately 1 ½-2 minutes or until melted completely, stirring after every 30 minutes.
4. Remove the bowl from microwave.
5. In the bowl of chocolate, add the coconut oil, flour and coconut milk and mix until a smooth mixture forms.
6. Set aside to cool completely.
7. In another medium-sized glass bowl, add honey, pumpkin puree, eggs and spices and whisk until blended thoroughly.
8. Add chocolate mixture in the bowl of egg mixture and mix until blended thoroughly.
9. Place the mixture into prepared cake pan evenly.
10. Bake for approximately 40 minutes.
11. Remove the cake pan from oven and place onto a wire rack for approximately 10 minutes.
12. Then invert the cake onto the wire rack to cool completely before frosting.
13. For frosting: in a medium-sized glass bowl, add all ingredients and mix until blended thoroughly.
14. Spread frosting over cake evenly and serve.

Nutritional Information per Serving:

Calories: 384
Fat: 30.4g
Net Carbohydrates: 14.9g
Carbohydrates: 19.9g
Fiber: 5g
Sugar: 10.3g

Protein: 6.8g
Sodium: 47mg

30 Days Meal Plan

Day 1

Breakfast: Avocado & Kale Smoothie
Lunch: Tempeh in Tomato Sauce
Dinner: Spicy Salmon Soup

Day 2

Breakfast: Microwave Oatmeal
Lunch: Shrimp Lettuce Wraps
Dinner: Ground Turkey with Cabbage

Day 3

Breakfast: Kale Scramble
Lunch: Squid with Veggies
Dinner: Black Beans & Veggie Chili

Day 4

Breakfast: Quinoa Bread
Lunch: Stuffed Zucchini
Dinner: Chicken & Tomato Curry

Day 5

Breakfast: Fruity Greens Smoothie Bowl
Lunch: Squid with Veggies
Dinner: Lentil & Potato Stew

Day 6

Breakfast: Tomato Omelet
Lunch: Carrot & Sweet Potato Soup
Dinner: Spicy Cod

Day 7

Breakfast: Pineapple Smoothie
Lunch: Potato Curry
Dinner: Ground Turkey with Greens

Day 8

Breakfast: Carrot Bread
Lunch: Quinoa in Tomato Sauce
Dinner: Cheesy salmon Parcel

Day 9

Breakfast: Banana Porridge
Lunch: Apple, Beet & Carrot Salad
Dinner: Chicken & Tomato Soup

Day 10

Breakfast: Carrot & Coconut Muffins
Lunch: Cauliflower Soup
Dinner: Tilapia with Veggies

Day 11

Breakfast: Fruity Yogurt Bowl
Lunch: Zucchini Lettuce Wraps
Dinner: Chicken Meatballs Curry

Day 12

Breakfast: Orange & Chia Smoothie
Lunch: Shrimp with Broccoli
Dinner: Red Kidney Beans Soup

Day 13

Breakfast: Pumpkin & Banana Waffles
Lunch: Broccoli Soup
Dinner: Turkey & Lentil Chili

Day 14

Breakfast: Kale Scramble
Lunch: Veggie Tortilla Wraps
Dinner: Salmon & Cabbage Soup

Day 15

Breakfast: Pumpkin Quinoa Porridge
Lunch: Asparagus & Spinach Curry
Dinner: Chicken with Pineapple

Day 16

Breakfast: Blueberry Smoothie Bowl
Lunch: Veggie Lettuce Wraps
Dinner: Tilapia Parcel

Day 17

Breakfast: Zucchini & Carrot Quiche
Lunch: Scallops with Veggies
Dinner: Chickpeas Chili

Day 18

Breakfast: Fruity Muffins
Lunch: Butternut Squash Soup
Dinner: Salmon with Peach

Day 19

Breakfast: Berries & Spinach Smoothie
Lunch: Mushroom & Corn Curry
Dinner: Ground Turkey & Cabbage Soup

Day 20

Breakfast: Mushroom & Arugula Frittata
Lunch: Pumpkin Soup
Dinner: Chicken & Beans Chili

Day 21

Breakfast: Pumpkin Chia Pudding
Lunch: Avocado & Tomato Sandwiches
Dinner: Salmon in Spicy Yogurt Sauce

Day 22

Breakfast: Crepes with Strawberry Sauce
Lunch: Chicken & Mango Tortilla Wraps
Dinner: Lentils & Veggie Soup

Day 23

Breakfast: Veggie Muffins
Lunch: Three Beans Chili
Dinner: Chicken, Jicama & Carrot Salad

Day 24

Breakfast: Banana Porridge
Lunch: Veggie Sandwiches
Dinner: Turkey with Bell Pepper & Asparagus

Day 25

Breakfast: Fruity Yogurt Bowl
Lunch: Zucchini Lettuce Wraps
Dinner: Chicken & Spinach Stew

Day 26

Breakfast: Quinoa Bread
Lunch: Veggies Gumbo
Dinner: Shrimp, Fruit & Bell Pepper Curry

Day 27

Breakfast: Cilantro Pancakes
Lunch: Berries & Watermelon Salad
Dinner: Chicken with Broccoli & Spinach

Day 28

Breakfast: Fruity Muffins
Lunch: Stuffed Zucchini
Dinner: Turkey & Squash Stew

peas & Squash Stew

Day 29

Breakfast: Overnight Fruity Chai Bowl
Lunch: Collard Greens & Seeds Salad
Dinner: Chicken Casserole

Day 30

Breakfast: Zucchini & Carrot Quiche
Lunch: Turkey Lettuce Wraps
Dinner: Chick

Conversion Chart

Mass

Imperial (ounces)	Metric (gram)
¼ ounce	7 grams
½ ounce	14 grams
1 ounce	28 grams
2 ounces	56 grams
3 ounces	85 grams
4 ounces	113 grams
5 ounces	141 grams
6 ounces	150 grams
7 ounces	198 grams
8 ounces	226 grams
9 ounces	255 grams
10 ounces	283 grams
11 ounces	311 grams
12 ounces	340 grams
13 ounces	368 grams
14 ounces	396 grams
15 ounces	425 grams
16 ounces/ 1 pound	455 grams

Cups & Spoon

Cups	Metric
¼ cup	60 millilitres
1/3 cup	80 millilitres
½ cup	120 millilitres
1 cup	240 millilitres

Spoon	Metric
¼ teaspoon	1¼ millilitres
½ teaspoon	2½ millilitres
1 teaspoon	5 millilitres
2 teaspoons	10 millilitres
1 tablespoon	20 millilitres

Liquid

Imperial	Metric
1 fluid ounce	30 millilitres
2 fluid ounces	60 millilitres
3½ fluid ounces	80 millilitres
2¾ fluid ounces	100 millilitres
4 fluid ounces	125 millilitres
5 fluid ounces	150 millilitres
6 fluid ounces	180 millilitres
7 fluid ounces	200 millilitres
8¾ fluid ounces	250 millilitres
10½ fluid ounces	310 millilitres
13 fluid ounces	375 millilitres
15 fluid ounces	430 millilitres
16 fluid ounces	475 millilitres
17 fluid ounces	500 millilitres
21½ fluid ounces	625 millilitres
26 fluid ounces	750 millilitres
35 fluid ounces	1 Liter
44 fluid ounces	1¼ Liters
52 fluid ounces	1½ Liters
70 fluid ounces	2 Liters
88 fluid ounces	2½ Liters

Conclusion

An anti-inflammatory diet should be an integral part of any comprehensive plan to reduce inflammation throughout the body. By simply introducing more vegetables, fruits and healthy fats while avoiding processed foods, one can start to take charge of the health of their body. Furthermore, ensuring adequate water intake has been shown to help clear out toxins that increase inflammation. Though this type of diet takes some effort and adjustments to become used to, the payoff is incredibly worthwhile as it leads to a healthier lifestyle overall.

Printed in Great Britain
by Amazon